CBS Examination Review 2005

All India PG Dental Entrance Examinations

for MDS

(with Explanations & References)

CBS Examination Review 2005

All India PG Dental Entrance Examinations

for MDS
(with Explanations & References)

Dr. Neeraj Gupta

CBS

CBS PUBLISHERS & DISTRIBUTORS

NEW DELHI • BANGALORE

ISBN : 81-239-1270-6

First Edition : 2005

Publishing Director : Vinod K. Jain

Published by :
Satish Kumar Jain for CBS Publishers & Distributors,
4596/1-A, 11 Darya Ganj, New Delhi - 110 002 (India)
E-mail : cbspubs@del3.vsnl.net.in
Website : http://www.cbspd.com

Branch Office :
2975, 17th Cross, K.R. Road,
Bansankari 2nd Stage, Bangalore - 560 070
Fax : 080-26771680 • E-mail : cbsbng@vsnl.net

Printed at :
Asia Printograph, Delhi

Dedicated to:

MAA SARASWATI DEVI,
My Parents, Brothers,
Other Family Members
&
My Teachers

PREFACE

With ever increasing students for competitions and a few seats of P.G. students, the competition for Entrance Examinations is becoming very difficult and hard to achieve the capability and capacity to get admissions without the extra ordinary efforts and meticulous understanding and confidence.

With increase in percentage of students who will not be able to fill in right answers for MCQs, it has become important that extensive and through going through the various questions to answer correctly is must. Today thorough knowledge of text, not only on the Dental subjects but also the basic subjects of Medical Science is imperative.

It is obvious that the trend of questions being repeated has been over and the advances in various subjects has created tremendous scope for putting-up questions on recent research which demands an extensive as well as broad base reading. Lastly, the questions are now being picked up not from the leading books like National Boards, Reeds or Bouchers but detailed questions pertaining to both MD/MS as well MDS examinations.

Further, the negative marking itself may become the greatest obstacle to come into the competition. The purpose of this book is not to create confusion to the competitors but to make the points of various books/subjects throughly clear, so that, as far as possible minimal errors are committed. There is not hesitation in recommending this book of MCQs for general reading as well as for thorough understanding to answer the questions correctly.

I would also like to thank Mr. Satish Kalra

and Punish Kumar for the help in composing this book. My appreciation also extends to Mr. S.K. Jain and his team from CBS Publishers and Distributors, New Delhi for bringing out this book.

Dr. NEERAJ GUPTA

ACKNOWLEDGEMENTS

There are a lot of names behind the successful completion of this book. First of all I would like to thank to "MAA SARASWATI DEVI" who gave me a power to do this herculean task. Then I would like to thank my friends and my seniors and other persons who inspired me and helps me in completionof this book. Dr. Amit Garg, Dr. Parveen Dahia, Dr. Rakesh Singhla, Dr. Sandeep Sabharwal, Dr. Amit Gandhi, Dr. Suresh Saini, Dr. Pankaj Sangwan, Dr. Pankaj Bansal, Dr. Anil Yadav, Dr. Deepak Chopra, Dr. Ajay Verma, Dr. Sumit Sharma, Dr. Sushil Sharma, Dr. Mukesh Rohilla, Dr. Balwant Rai, Dr. Rajesh Birla, Dr. Rajesh Singla, Dr. Ajit Rohilla, Dr. Vinod Dhaniya, Dr. Pardeep Sabharwal, Dr. Hansraj Saini, Mrs. Babita Garg, Mr. Satish Popli, Mr. Rajesh Gautam and Mr. Raj and the teaches of Govt. Dental College, Rohtak who support and guide to write this book.

(Dr. Neeraj Gupta)

REFERENCES

1. **Anatomy** - B.D. Chaurasia, Gen. Anatomy B.D. Chaurasia, Snells, A.K. Halim for Dental Students.
2. **Physiology** - Ganong, Chaudhari, R.L. Bijlani, R.K. Marya
3. **Biochemistry** - Harper, Lipincott, H. Lal
4. **Microbiology** - Ananthnarayan, D.R. Arora
5. **Pathology** - Robbins
6. **Pharmacology** - K.D. Tripathi, Katzung, Naresh Khanna
7. **Dental Anatomy Histology** - Orbans, Tencate
8. **Surgery** - S. Das, Bailey and Love, Watkinson, Shenoy
9. **Medicine** - Harrison, Khosla
10. **Oral Pathology** - Shafer
11. **Preventive and Community Dentistry** - Satish Chandra, Joseph John, Sobenpeter
12. **Radiology** - Vimal Sikri, Parmod John R., White and Pharoah, Walter and Miller
13. **Oral Surgery** - Vinod Kapoor, Malamed Handbook of Medical Emergency Malamed handbook of local anaesthesia.
14. **Periodontics** - Carranza
15. **Pedodontics** - Shobha Tandon, Damle, Mcdonald
16. **Operative** - Sturdevent, Vimal Sikri, Gilmore
17. **Endodontics** - Ingle, Cohen Burns, Vimal Sikri
18. **Orthodontics** - Rani, Bhalajhi, Profitt, Jeffery Okesson
19. **Prosthodontics** - Bernarld Levine, Boucher, Hertwell, Nallaswamy, Tylman, Rosenstiel, Misch, Schillinberg
20. **ENT** - Bhargava, Dhingra, Marvin P. Fried
21. **Forensic Medicine** - Parikh, Reddy, Krishan Vij, V. Subhrahmanyam
22. **SPM** - Park and Park
23. **Biostatics** - NMS Series, High yield biostatics
24. **Paediatrics** - O.P. Ghai, Dutta.
25. **Psychiatry** - M.S. Bhatia, Niraj Ahuja
26. **Anaesthesia** - Ajay Yadav

CONTENTS

Q.1. The following statement concerning chorda tympani nerve are true except that it:

1. Carries secretomotor fibres to submandibular gland.
2. Join lingual nerve in infratemporal fossa.
3. Is a branch of facial nerve.
4. Contains postganglionic parasympathetic fibres.

Ans. (4). Contains post ganglionic parasympathetic fibres *(B.D. Chaurasia, Vol. III, 3rd ed. P. 113)*.

- Chorda tympani arises in the vertical part of facial canal about 6 mm above stylomastoid foramen.
- It runs upward and forward in a bony canal.
- It enters the middle ear and runs forward in close relation to the tympanic membrane.
- It leaves the middle ear by passing through petrotympanic fissure.
- It passes medial to spine of sphenoid and enters the infratemporal fossa. Here it joins the lingual nerve through which it is distributed.
- It carries Preganglionic secretomotor fibre to the submandibular ganglion for supply of the submandibular and sublingual salivary glands and taste fibre from anterior 2/3rd of the tongue.

Q.2. Palatine aponeurosis:

1. Tendon of levator veli palatine muscle.
2. Tendon of tensor veli palatine muscle.
3. A part of musculus uvulae.
4. A modification of palatal periosteum.

Ans. (2). Tendon of Tensor veli palatine muscle *(B.D. Chaurasia, Vol. III, 3rd ed. P. 179, 180).*

The palatine aponeurosis (which is the flattened tendon of the tensor palati) forms the fibrous basis of the palate. Near the median plane the aponeurosis split to enclose the musculus uvulae.

Q.3. All of the following physiological processes occur during the growth at the epiphyseal plate except:

1. Proliferation and hypertrophy.
2. Calcification and ossification.
3. Vasculogenesis and erosion.
4. Replacement of red bone marrow with yellow marrow.

Ans. (4). Replacement of red bone marrow with yellow marrow. *(General Anatomy, B.D. Chaurasia 3rd ed., P. 33).*

Epiphyseal plate under go changes with ages, which are:

1. Proliferation and hypertrophy resulting in lengthening of a long bone.
2. Calcification and ossification occur which cause fusion of epiphysis after which no linear growth occurs.
3. Vasculogenesis and erosion resulting in anastomosis between epiphyseal and metaphyseal arteries after fusion of epiphysis.

No bone marrow occur in epiphyseal plate, so no replacement of red bone marrow with yellow bone marrow.

Q.4. Which of the following is the normal arrangement of lingual nerve and vessels in the tongue from medial to lateral?

1. Nerve, Artery, Vein
2. Artery, Nerve, Vein
3. Vein, Artery, Nerve
4. Nerve, Artery

Ans. (2). Artery, Nerve, Vein *(Snells 7th ed. P. 845, A.K. Halm for dental students 1st ed., P. 178).*

For this question there is no direct written references. But on the above given page of referred book see the diagram that

– Deep lingual artery lie medial side

– Deep lingual vein lie lateral side

Lingual nerve lie between these two structures i.e. between deep lingual artery and deep lingual vein.

So the answer is Artery, Nerve, Vein.

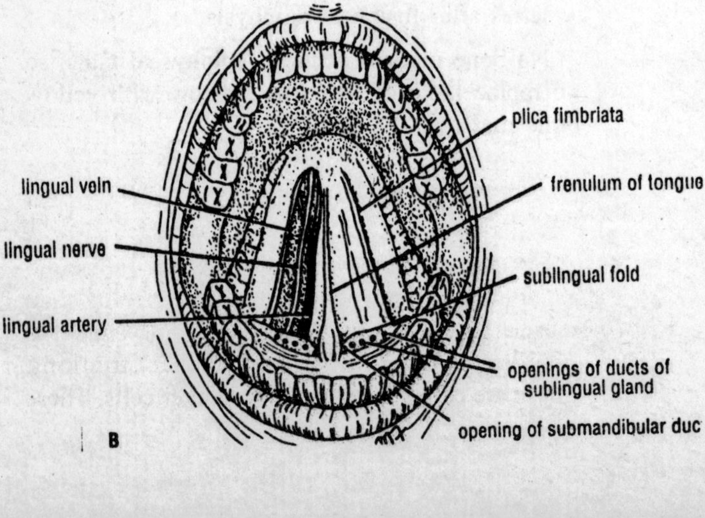

Q.5. SA node act as a pacemaker of the heart because of the fact that it:

1. is capable of generating impulse spontaneously.
2. Has rich sympathetic innervations.
3. Has poor cholinergic innervations.
4. Generate impulse at the highest rate.

Ans. (4). Generate impulse at the highest rate *(Harrison 15th ed., P. 1284).*

- SA node is normally the dominant cardiac pacemaker because its intrinsic discharge rate is the highest of all the potential cardiac pacemakers.
- Its responsiveness to alteration in autonomic nervous system is responsible for normal acceleration of heart rate during exercise and the slowing that occurs during rest and sleep.
- Increase in sinus rate is normally result from an increase in sympathetic tone acting via ß adrenergic receptors and/or decrease in parasympathetic tone acting via muscarinic receptors.

More about SA node:

Location: on the posterior aspect of heart at the junction of the superior vena cava (SVC) with right atrium (i.e. free border of the RA appendix).

Dimensions: length 15 m, width 2 mm, Thickness 1 mm.

Structure: Highly vascular, consist of thin, elongated muscle fibres (approx. 1/3 the size of heart muscle fibre), rich in glycogen and mitochondria, fusiform in shape with longitudinal striations. These are called P-cells or pacemaker cells. These fibres normally can generate and discharge impulse more rapidly than any other pacemaker tissue and their rate of discharge determines the rate at which the heart beats. That is why SAN is called the cardiac pacemaker.

Innervation: It develops from structures on the right side of the embryo that is why, in adults, SAN is innervated by right vagus nerve. It also receive sympathetic nerve fibres predominantly of right side from cervical sympathetic ganglia via the cardiac nerves. SA node conduction speed is 0.05 m/sec.

Q.6. CO_2 is primarily transported in the arterial blood as:

1. Dissolved CO_2
2. Carbonic acid
3. Carbamino haemoglobin
4. Bicarbonate.

Ans. (4). Bicarbonate *(Ganong 20th ed., P. 648).*

- 78% is transported as Bicarbonate (43.8 ml/dl)
- 11% is transported as Carbamino compound (2.6 ml/dl) and
- 11% is transported as dissolved in Plasma (2.6 ml/dl).

Something more:

- Amount of oxygen that enters body/min = 250 ml/min.
- Amount of CO_2 excreted by lungs/min = 200 ml/min (this comes out to be = 288 L/day).
- Chloride shifts takes about: 1 sec.
- Haematocrit of venous blood is greater (by 3%) than that of arterial blood.
- PH of venous blood is: Lower than that of arterial blood (7.36 in place of 7.40 in Arterial blood).

Q.7. In which of the following a reduction in arterial oxygen tension occurs:

1. Anaemia
2. Copoisoning
3. Moderate Exercise
4. Hypoventilation

Ans. (4). Hypoventilation *(Ganong 20th ed., P. 660, 666, Chaudhary 3rd ed., P. 143).*

Type	Mechanism	PaO_2	PaO_2	O_2 content
Hypoxic hypoxia	Decreased partial pressure of oxygen in arterial blood - High altitude (hypoventilation) - Respiratory disease	↓	↓	↓
Anemic hypoxia	Decreased oxygen carrying capacity of blood - Low Hb - CO poisoning	±	±	↓
Stagnant ischemic hypoxia	O_2 content of blood is exhausted due to reduction in blood velocity - Cardiogenic shock	±	±	±
Histologic hypoxia	Tissues cannot make use of available oxygen - Inhibition of Cytochrome oxidase system - Cyanide (HCN) poisoning	±	±	±

- Arterial O_2 tension (PaO_2) 95 ± 5 mmHg
- Arterial CO_2 tension ($PaCO_2$) 40 ± 2 mmHg
- Arterial O_2 saturation 97 ± 2%
- Arterial blood pH 7.4 ± 0.2
- Dead space volume 2 ml/kg body wt.

Q.8. The blood cells responsible for humoral immunity are:

1. T-cells
2. B-cells
3. No cells only antibodies
4. Mostly B-cells sometimes T-cells

Ans. (2). Mostly B cells sometimes T cell *(Ganong 19th ed., P. 502)*.

When an antigen enters the body it is ingested by macrophage and partially digested. This processed antigen with the macrophage then binds to receptor. On T lymphocytes activating helper T cells (T_4 cells). The T_4 cells then activate B lymphocyte causing them to proliferate and transform in to memory B cells and plasma cells.

Q.9. The cell component that is genetically continuous from one cell generation to the next:

1. Nuclear membrane
2. Golgi complex
3. Central bodies
4. Chromatin

Ans. (4). Chromatin *(Chaudhari 2nd ed., P. 3).*

When a cell is at rest, its DNA molecule in combination with some protein, are seen in the light microscope as dark irregular clumps of material and are known as chromatin. During cell division, however they become coiled and condensed and are seen as rod shaped bodies called chromosome and carry information from generation to generation.

(Chaudhari)

Read text below:

Chromatin (Flemming 1879) – It is a fibrous hereditary material formed by DNA histone complex. Chromatin fibre are of two types:

1. Euchromatin
2. Heterochromatin

- Replication occur late in heterochromatin. Constitutive heterochromatin occurs in all cell and in all stages including chromosome.
- Facultative heterochromatin is formed in certain cells to inactivate certain genes.
- Once X chromosome in human female become facultative heterochromatic during early embryogenesis. It become normal in oocytes.
- Barr body develop due to it. Chromatin is actually folded nucleosome (DNA & histone) containing DNA chains.

- During nuclear division chromatin fibres fold variously to produce chromosome.
- Base pairs constitute nucleic acid which carry genetic information from generation to generation.

Q.10. Adam stokes syndrome is caused due to:

1. Atrial fibrillation
2. Atrial extrasystole
3. Complete AV block.
4. Ventilation fibrillation.

Ans. (3). Complete AV block *(R.L. Bijlani, 3rd ed., P. 180; Ganong 19th Ed., P. 529).*

Third Degree or Complete Heart Block:

When AV node fails to conduct any atrial impulse to the ventricles, the condition is called third degree or complete heart block. Then the ventricles start beating at their own rhythm, called the idioventricular rhythm, which is only 20 to 40 beats per min. Therefore, the ECG shows complete desynchronisation of P and QRST waves. P waves are more numerous than QRST waves. Therefore a P wave may be seen before, during or after a QRST wave. Sometimes P cannot be seen, as it gets masked by strong QRS complexes. Mutual interaction of P and QRS may produce many bizarre wave forms. However, if this condition occurs suddenly, before the idioventricular rhythm gets established, heart may stop for a few seconds leading to dizziness or fainting. When the heart stops longer, the condition is known as Stokes-Adams syndrome. Immediate cardiac massage may stimulate idioventricular rhythm and save the patient. Complete heart block may be due to ischaemia or infarction of AV nodal region.

Q.11. Distribution of blood flow is mainly regulated by the:

1. Arteries
2. Arterioles
3. Capillaries
4. Venules

Ans. (2). Arterioles *(Muthayya 3rd ed., P. 354, Ganong 19th ed., P. 550).*

Arterioles: The small arteries divide and subdivide and form arterioles. The walls of these are composed entirely of smooth muscle fibres and by a layer of endothelial cells and sheathed by adventitia. The muscle fibres are supplied by excitatory and inhibitory vasomotor nerves. These arterioles act as stop-cocks which control the blood flow from arteries into the capillaries and help in appropriate distribution of blood to various tissue according to their needs. These convert the pulsatile arterial blood flow into a non-pulsatile flow through the capillaries. The arterioles are the main sites of peripheral resistance. Hence there are known as "resistance vessels".

Q.12. The first physiological response to high environmental temperature is:

1. Sweating
2. Vasodilation
3. Decreased heat production
4. Non-shivering thermogenesis

Ans. (2). Vasodilation *(R.L. Bijlani 3rd ed., P. 318-320, Ganong 19th ed., P. 241).*

Factors affecting heat balance

Heat gain	Heat loss
<u>Increased heat production</u>	<u>Increased heat dissipation</u>
1. Shivering	1. Cutaneous vasodilation
2. Neurohumoral stimulation of metabolic rate	2. Sweating
3. Exercise	3. Panting
4. Thermic effect of feeding	4. Air movement
	5. Cooler environment
6. Increased surface area	6. Increase surface area
<u>Decreased heat loss</u>	<u>Decreased heat conservation</u>
1. Cutaneous vasoconstriction	1. Reduced insulation (clothing/fur)
2. Increased insulation (Clothing/fur)	
3. Reduced air movement	
4. Warmer environment	
5. Reduced surface area	

Q.13. A simple bacterial test for mutagenic carcinoges is:

1. Ames test
2. Redox test
3. Bacteriophage
4. Gene splicing

Ans. (1). Ames test *(U. Satyanarayan 1st ed., P. 606, Harper 25th ed., P. 789).*

Ames assay:

This is a laboratory test to check the carcinogenicity of chemicals. Ames assay employs the use of a special mutant strain of bacterium namely salmonella typhinurium (His). This organism cannot synthesise histidine hence the same should be supplied in the medium for its growth. Addition of chemical carcinogens causes mutation (reverse mutation) restoring the ability of bacteria to synthesise histidine. By detecting the strain of salmonella (His+) in the colonies of agar plates, the chemical mutogens can be identified. The Ames assay can detect about 90% of the chemical carcinogens.

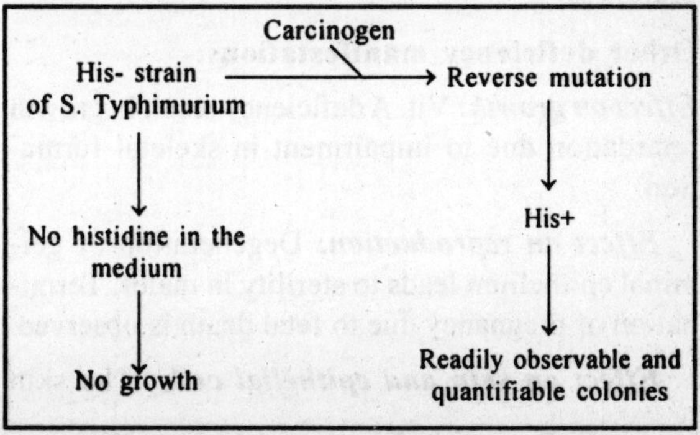

Q.14. Vitamin A:

1. Is water soluble
2. Deficiency cause impaired vision
3. Maintain normal plasma calcium levels.
4. Is required for formation of clotting factors.

Ans. (2). Deficiency cause impaired vision *(U. Satyanarayan 1st ed., P. 120).*

Vitamin A deficiency:

Night blindness (nyctalopia) is one of the earliest symptoms of vitamin A deficiency.

Xeropthalmia: Severe deficiency of vitamin A leads to xeropthalmia. This is characterised by dryness in conjunctiva and cornea keratinisation of epithelial cells. In certain areas of conjunctiva, white triangular plaques known as Bitot's spots are seen.

Keratomalacia: If xeropthalmia persists for a long time, corneal ulceration and degeneration occur. This result in destruction of cornea, a condition referred to as Keratomalacia causing total blindness.

Other deficiency manifestations:

Effect on growth: Vit. A deficiency result in growth retardation due to impairment in skeletal formation.

Effect on reproduction: Degeneration of germinal epithelium leads to sterility in males. Termination of pregnancy due to fetal death is observed.

Effect on skin and epithelial cells: The skin

become rough and dry vit. A def. is associated with formation of urinary stones. The plasma level of retinal binding protein is decreased in vit.A deficiency.

***Hypervitaminosis A*:** Excessive consumption of vit.A lead to toxicity. The symptoms of hypervitaminosis A include dermatitis (drying and redness of skin), enlargement of liver, skeletal decalcification, tenderness of long bones, loss of weight, irritating, loss of hair, joint pains etc. The subjects have constant headache due to raised intracranial pressure.

Q.15. Both vitamin K and C are involved in:

1. The synthesis of clotting factors
2. Post translational modifications
3. Antioxidant mechanisms
4. The microsomal hydroxylation reactions

Ans. (2). Post translational modifications *(Harper 25th ed., P. 640, 649, 697).*

Vitamin C is required for post translational modification of proline and lysine in collagen synthesis. Vitamin K is required for post translational modification of glutamate residues for generation of clotting factors.

Thus both undergo post translational modification is the correct statement.

- Only vit C helps in conversion of proline to hydroxyproline and not vit K.
- Only Vit. K is involved in coagulation cascade (helps in generation of biological active clotting factors).

Q.16. Of the following minerals the highest amount found in human body is:

1. Sodium
2. Calcium
3. Phosphorus
4. Iron

Ans. (2). Calcium *(U. Satyanarayan 1st ed., P. 449).*

- Calcium constitute about 2% of body weight
- Calcium is the most abundant among the minerals in the body.
- The total content of calcium in an adult man is about 1–1.5 kg.
- 99% of it is present in bones and teeth.
- 1% of the calcium found outside the skeletal tissue, performs a wide variety of functions.

Biochemical functions:

1. Development of bone and teeth
2. Muscle contraction
3. Blood coagulation
4. Nerve transmission
5. Membrane integrity and permeability
6. Activation of enzymes
7. Calmodulin mediated action of Ca^{2+}
8. Calcium as intracellular messenger
9. Release of hormones
10. Secretory process
11. Contact inhibition
12. Action on heart

Dietary requirement: Adult men and women - 800 mg/day.

Women during pregnancy - 15 g/day.

Lactation and menopause

Children (1-18 yrs) - 0.8-1.2 g/day

Infants (<1 year) - 300-500 mg/day

Plasma Calcium: The normal conc. of plasma or serum Ca is 9-11 mg/dl (4.5-5.5 mEq/L).About half of this (5 mg/dl) is in ionised form which is functionally the most active. At least 1 mg/dl serum Ca is found in association with citrate and phosphate. Other half of serum Ca (4-5 mg/dl) is bound to proteins, mostly albumin and to a lesser extent globulin.

Q.17. The membrane protein, clathrin is involved in:

1. Cell motility
2. Receptor-mediated endocytosis
3. Exocytosis
4. Cell shape

Ans. (2). Receptor-mediated endocytosis *(Harper 25th ed., P. 530, Ganong 20th ed., P. 27).*

Endocytosis:

- The process by which cells take up large molecules is called endocytosis.
- Endocytotic vesicles are generated when segments of the plasma membrane invaginate, enclosing a minute volume of extracellular fluid and its content. The vesicle then pinches off as the fusion of plasma membrane seals the neck of the vesicle at the original site of invagination.
- There are two general types of endocytosis:
  - Phagocytosis
  - Pinocytosis

Phagocytosis:

- Involves ingestion of large particles such as viruses, bacteria, cells or debris.
- Phagocytosis occurs only in specialized cells such as macrophages and granulocytes.

Pinocytosis:

- It is a property of all cells
- It is a cellular uptake of fluid and fluid contents.
- Pinocytosis is of two types:

(a) ***Fluid phase pinocytosis:*** is a non-selective

process in which the uptake of a solute is simply proportionate to its concentration in the surrounding extracellular fluid:

(b) ***Absorptive pinocytosis:*** is a receptor mediated selective process primarily responsible for the uptake of macromolecules. The vesicles formed during absorptive pinocytosis are derived from invagination (pits) that are coated on the cytoplasmic side with a filamentous material. In many systems, clathrin is the filamentous material. For e.g. LDL is internalized by means of coated pits containing the LDL receptors.

Q.18. The amino acid residue having an imino side chain is:

1. Lysine
2. Histidine
3. Tyrosine
4. Proline

Ans. (4). Proline *(U. Satyanarayan 1st ed., P. 50, Harper 25th ed., P. 28).*

More about proline:

- Proline containing pyrrolidine ring is a unique amino acid, it has an imino group (=NH) instead of amino group. Hydroxyproline is proline derivative found in proteins.
- Proline is never found in α-helix.
- Proline is oxidised to pyrroline-5-carboxylate which undergoes a non-enzymatic conversion to glutamate-5-semialdehyde.
- The latter is converted to glutamate and then transaminated to α-ketoglutarate. The five carbons of proline are converted to α-ketoglutarate.
- ***Hyperprolinemia type I*** – is due to a defect in the enzyme proline oxidase (Proline dehydrogenase).
- ***Hyperprolinemia type II*** – associated with hydroxyproline metabolism.

Amino acid	**Special group present**
Cysteine	Sulfahydryl
Cystine	Disulfide
Methionine	Thioether
Aspartic acid	ß carboxyl
Asparagine	Amide

Glutamic acid	γ carboxyl
Glutamine	Amide
Lysine	E-Amino
Arginine	Guanidino
Histidine	Imidazole
Phenylamine	Benzene or phenyl
Tyrosine	Phenol
Tryptophan	Indole
Proline	Pyrrolidine
	Glutamine

Imino acids

- Proline

Aromatic amino acid

- Histidine
- Phenyalanine
- Tyrosine
- Tryptophan

Basic amino acid

- Arginine
- Lysine
- Histidine

Acidic amino acid

- Aspartic
- Aspartate
- Glutamic acid

Sulphur containing AA

- Cysteine
- Methionine

Q.19. Enzyme that move a molecular group from one molecule to another are known as:

1. Ligases
2. Oxido-reductases
3. Transferases
4. Dipeptidases

Ans. (3). Transferases *(Lippincott 2nd ed., P. 47)*.

Transferase are enzymes that catalyses the transfer of functional groups from one molecule to another. The six major class of enzymes.

1. **Oxidoreductase:** Catalyse oxidation reduction reaction.
2. **Transferase:** Catalyses transfer of S, N or P containing groups.
3. **Hydrolases:** Catalyses cleavage bonds by addition of water eg. Peptidase which degrade peptide to free amino acids.
4. **Lyases:** Catalyses cleavage of C-C, C-S and certain C-N bonds.
5. **Isomerase:** Catalyse racemization of optical or geometric isomers.
6. **Ligase:** Catalyse formation of bonds between C&O, S, N coupled to hydrolysis of high energy phosphates.

Q.20. All of the following are true about manifestations of Vitamin E deficiency, except:

1. Haemolytic Anaemia
2. Posterior column abnormalities
3. Cerebellar ataxia
4. Autonomic dysfunction.

Ans. (4). Autonomic dysfunction *(Harrison 15th ed., P. 467).*

Deficiency of Vit. E:

- Dietary deficiency of vit.E does not exist. Vit.E deficiency is seen only in severe and prolonged malabsorptive disease. Such as cardiac disease or after small intestinal resection.
- Children with cystic fibrosis or prolonged cholestatis may develop vit.E deficiency characterised by areflexia and haemolytic anaemia.
- Children with abetalipoproteinemia cannot absorb or transport vit. E and become deficient quite rapidly.
- Vit.E deficiency cause axonal degeneration of large myelinated axons and results in posterior column and spinocerebellar symptoms.
- Peripheral neuropathy is initially characterised by areflexia, with progression to an ataxic gait and by decreased vibration and position sensations.
- Ophthalmoplegia, skeletal myopathy, pigmented retinopathy occur due to vit.E deficiency.

The laboratory diagnosis of vitamin E deficiency is made on the basis of low blood levels of α-tocopherol <5 μg/ml or < 0.8 mg of α-tocopherol per gram of total lipids.

Toxicity of Vit. E: High dose of vit. E (>800 mg/d) may reduce platelet aggregation and interfere with vit. K metabolism and are therefore contraindicated in patients taking coumadin. Nausea, flatulence, diarrhoea have been reported at dose >1 g/d.

Q.21 Vitamin B_{12} deficiency can give rise to all of the following except:

1. Myelopathy
2. Optic atrophy
3. Peripheral neuropathy
4. Myopathy

Ans. (4). Myopathy *(Harrison 15th ed., P. 677, 2432).*

Deficiency of vit. B_{12} cause:

1. Haematologic manifestation:

Anaemic symptoms (megaloblastic anaemia)

- Vertigo
- Tinnitus
- Light headedness
- Palpitations
- Angina

2. Gastrointestinal manifestation:

- Sore tongue
- Smooth, beefy red tongue
- Anorexia
- Moderate weight loss
- Diarrhoea
- Glossitis

3. Neurologic manifestations:

- Demyelination
- Optic atrophy, (Posterior and lateral tracts involvement)
- Subacute combined degeneration of spinal cord (Myelopathy)
- Peripheral neuropathy
- Axonal degeneration
- Eventual neuronal death

- Numbness and paresthesia in the extremities (Earliest neurologic manifestation)
- Weakness of ataxia
- Sphincter disturbance
- Reflexes may be diminished or increased
- Romberg and Babinksi sign may be positive
- Vibration senses diminished.

The diagnosis is confirmed by the finding of a low serum B_{12} concentration elevated level of homocysteine and methylmalonic acid in uncertain cases and a positive schilling test.

Myopathy is caused by vitamin D deficiency.

Q.22. Golgi bodies are responsible for:

1. Synthesis of polypeptides
2. Formation of glycoproteins only
3. Modification and sorting of glycoproteins
4. Lipid and steroid synthesis.

Ans. (3). Modification and sorting of glycoproteins (*Harper 25th ed., P.9, U. Satyanarayan 1st ed., P. 4*).

Golgi apparatus:

Marker - Galactosyl transferase.

Major function:

1. Intracellular sorting of proteins
2. Glycosylation reaction
3. Sulfation reactions - *(Harper 25th ed.)*

Golgi apparatus:

Dictyosome constitute Golgi complex. The newly synthesised proteins are handed over to the golgi apparatus which catalyse the addition of carbohydrate, lipids or sulfate moieties to the proteins. These chemical modifications are necessary for the transport of proteins across the plasma membrane.

(U. Satyanarayan)

Q.23. Fluoride, used in the collection of blood samples for glucose estimation inhibits the enzymes:

1. Glucokinase
2. Hexokinase
3. Enolase
4. Glucose-6-Phosphatase

Ans. (3). Enolase *(Harper 25th ed., P. 194).*

$$\text{2 Phosphoglycerate} \xrightarrow[\text{Fluoride Inhibitor}]{\text{Enolase Mg/Mn}} \text{Phosphoenol-pyrovate} + H_2O$$

Enolase is inhibited by fluoride: This can be made use of when it is required to prevent glycolysis in blood prior to estimation of glucose.

(Harper 25th ed.)

Read text below:

Inhibitors of Metabolic Pathway

Kreb cycle	Glycolysis
Fluoroacetate inhibits Aconitase $\text{Citrate} \xrightarrow[\text{Aconitase}]{} \text{isocitrate}$	Iodoacetate inhibits glycoaldehyde 3 phosphate dehydrogenase Glycoaldehyde 3-P dehydrogenase $\xrightarrow{\text{G-3PD}} \text{1,3 Phosphoglycerate}$
Arsenite (α Ketoglutarate) inhibits α K-6 dehydrogenase → Succinyl CoA	Fluoride inhibits enolase.
Malonate inhibits succinate dehydrogenase $\text{Succinate} \xrightarrow[\text{Succinate dehydrogenase}]{} \text{Fumrate}$	$\text{2 Phosphoglycerate} \xrightarrow{\text{Enolase}} \text{Phosphopenol pyruvate}$

Q.24. The protective effect of breast milk are known to be associated with:

1. IgM antibodies
2. Lysozyme
3. Mast cell
4. IgA antibodies

Ans. (4). IgA antibodies *(O.P. Ghai 5th ed., P. 63,126, Dutta 5th ed., P. 484).*

IgA secretory antibodies exerts its protective action by preventing bacterial contact to epithelial cells surface thus preventing gastrointestinal infections.

Breast milk contains a number of protective factors which include immunoglobulins. Secretary IgA, macrophages lymphocytes, lactoferrin, lysozyme, bifidus factor, interferon.

Nutritive value:

- Carbohydrate — Lactose (6–7 g/dl) ⟶ enhance growth of lactobacili in intestine, absorption of Ca.
- Galactose ⟶ Form galactocerebrosides.
- Proteins ⟶ 0.9-1.1 g/dl (Lactalbumin, Lactoglobulin).
- Amino acid ⟶Taurine.
- Cysteine ⟶ Necessary for neurotransmission and neuromodulation.
- Fat ⟶ have polyunsaturated fatty acids necessary for myelination of nervous system.
- Omega 2, 6 ⟶ Long chain fatty acids ⟶ formation of prostaglandins and cholesterol.
- Vitamins, minerals.
- Water, electrolytes.

Q.25. Osteoclast are inhibited by:

1. Parathyroid hormone
2. Calcitonin
3. 1,25-dihydroxy cholecalciferol
4. Tumour necrosis factor.

Ans. (2). Calcitonin *(Ganong 20th ed., P. 373).*

Stimulation of osteoblasts is caused by following hormone.

1. PTH
2. TNF
3. T3,T4
4. 1,25 dihydroxy cholecalciferol

Inhibition of osteoblast:

1. Corticosteroids

Stimulation of osteoclast:

1. PTH
2. 1,25 dihydroxy cholecalciferol
3. IL-6, IL-11

Inhibition of osteoclast:

1. Estrogens
2. Calcitonin
3. PGE2
4. TGF-B

Q.26. All of the following hormones have cell surface receptors except:

1. Adrenaline
2. Growth hormone
3. Insulin
4. Thyroxine

Ans. (4). Thyroxine *(Harper 25th ed., P. 535).*

Cell Membrane Receptors	**Cytoplasmic Receptors**	**Nuclear Receptors**
CAMP Pathway	(Steroid hormones)	(Thyroid hormones)
Adrenaline	Glucocorticoids	Thyroid hormones
Gulcagon	Mineralocorticoids	Thyroxin
TSH, FSH, LH	Estrogens	Tri-Iodothyronine
PTH, Calcitonin, ACTH	Progestins	
ID_3/DAG generation		
Vasopressin/oxytocin		
Tyrosine kinase reaction		
Insulin/Growth hormone		

Q.27. Desmodont is another name for:

1. The tooth with one wall pocket
2. Tooth with three walled pocket
3. Periodontal ligament
4. Dehiscence

Ans. (3). Periodontal ligament *(Orbans 11th ed., P. 204, Jablonski dictionary).*

Periodontal ligament have been described by a number of terms. These are:

1. Desmodont
2. Gomphosis
3. Pericementum
4. Dental periosteum
5. Alveodental ligament
6. Periodontal membrane

Periodontal membrane and periodontal ligament are now most commonly used.

The periodontal ligament has a number of functions which include:

1. Attachment and support
2. Nutrition
3. Synthesis and resorption
4. Proprioception

Q.28. The average diameter of coronal deutinal tubule near the pulp is:

1. 0.2-0.5 microns
2. 2-3 microns
3. 0.2-0.3 microns
4. 4-7 micorns

Ans. (2).2-3 microns *(Orbans 11th ed., P. 107, 108)*.

- The course of a dentinal tubules follows a gentle curve in the crown, less so in the root where it resembles a gentle S shape. Starting at right angles from the pulpal surfaces, the first convexity of this doubly curved course is directed toward the apex of the tooth.
- The tubule end perpendicular to the dentinoenamel and dentinocementum junction.
- The tubules are longer than the dentin is thick because they curve through dentin. The dentin ranges in thickness from 3 to 10 mm or more.
- They are larger in diameter near the pulpal cavity (3-4 μm) and smaller at their outer ends (1 μm).
- The ratio between no of tubules per unit area on the pulpal and outer surface of dentin is about 4:1.
- Near the pulpal surface of the dentin the number per square millimeter varys between 50000 and 90000.
- There are more tubules per unit area in the crown than in root.
- The ratio between outer and inner surface of dentin is about 5:1.

Q.29. In which part of oral cavity mucous membrane is the thinnest:

1. Soft palate
2. Labial mucosa
3. Floor of mouth
4. Buccal mucosa.

Ans. (3). Floor of mouth *(Ten Cate 5th ed., P. 377).*

Floor of mouth: Very thin (100 μm), non-keratinised, stratified squamous epithelium.

Soft palate: Thin (150 μm), non-keratinised stratified squamous epithelium.

Labial and buccal mucosa: Very thick (500 μm), non keratinised, stratified squamous epithelium.

Gingiva: Thick (250 μm), orthokeratinised or parakeratinised, stratified squamous epithelium often showing stippled surface.

Q.30. What is the thickness of the layer of prismless enamel found in primary teeth?

1. 25 µm
2. 50 µm
3. 75 µm
4. 100 µm

Ans. (1).25 µm *(Orbans 11th ed., P. 62).*

A relatively structureless layer of enamel approximately 30 µm thick has been described in 70% of permanent teeth and all deciduous teeth. This structureless enamel is found least often over the cusp tip and most commonly toward the cervical area of enamel surface. In this surface layer no prism outline are visible, and all the apatite crystal are parallel to one another and perpendicular to striae of Reitzus. It is somewhat more heavily mineralized than the bulk of enamel beneath other microscopic details observed on outer enamel surfaces of newly erupted teeth are Perikymata, rod ends, cracks (lamellae)

In above explanation 30 µm is the answer but in question 25 µm is near to 30 µm. So answer is 25 µm.

Q.31. The most common pathogens responsible for nosocomial pneumonias in the ICU are:

1. Gram positive organisms
2. Gram negative organisms
3. Mycoplasma
4. Viral infection

Ans. (2). Gram negative organism
(Ananthnarayan 6th ed., P. 588, Robbins 7th ed., P. 752, Harrison 15th ed., P. 858).

- Multiple resistant staphylococus aureus and gram negative bacilli are common pathogen responsible for nosocomial pneumonia.

(Ananthnarayan 6th ed.)

Remember:

- MC nosocomial infections ⟶ UTI
- MC organism causing nosocomial UTI ⟶ Proteus
- MC organism causing nosocomial pneumonia ⟶ Pseudomonas aeruginosa

Nosocomial pneumonia is common in patient with severe underlying disease, immunosuppression, prolonged antibiotic therapy or invasive devices such as intravascular catheters. Patient on mechanical ventilation are at particularly high risk. Gram negative rods (Enterobacteriaceae and pseudomonas species) and staphylococcus aureus are the most common isolates.

(Robbins 7th ed.)

- The major organism of concern in nosocomial pneumonia are gram negative aerobic bacteria. Pseudomonas aeruginosa was the most common isolate in the NNIS survey of ICUs with a frequency of 21%.

Staph aureus was next most common at 20%. Actinobacter has become a more common pathogen in ventilator associated pneumonia virus such as respiratory synctial virus, adenovirus are receiving increased attention as etiologic agents of nosocomial pneumonia in both adults and children.

(Harrison 15th ed.)

Q.32. Virus can be isolated from clinical samples by cultivation in the following except:

1. Tissue culture
2. Embryonated egg
3. Animals
4. Chemically defined media

Ans. (4). Chemically defined media *(Ananthnarayan 6th ed., P. 407).*

As virus are obligate intracellular parasites, they can not be grown on any inanimate culture medium. Three methods are employed for the cultivation of viruses.

1. **Inoculation in animals:** The earliest method for the cultivation of viruses causing human disease was inoculation into human volunteers for their pioneering work on yellow fever.

- Monkeys were used for isolation of the poliovirus by Landsteiner and popper.
- The use of white mice pioneered by Theiler extended the scope of animal inoculation greatly.
- Infant (suckling mice) are very susceptible to coxsakie and arboviruses.
- Animal inoculation is also used for the study of pathogeneis, immune response, epidemiology, oncogenesis.

2. **Embryonated egg:** Inoculation on the chorioallantoic membrane produces visible lesion (Pocks).

- Inoculation in to allantoic cavity provides a rich yield of influenza and somspara myxovirus.
- Chick embryo vaccine in routine use are the

yellow fever (17D Strain) and rabies (Flury strain)

3. **Cell culture:** Three types of tissue culture are available:

- Organ culture
- Explant culture
- Cell culture

***Some cell cultures used are*:**

- Primary cell culture
- Diploid cell strains
- Continuous cell lines

Q.33. Type I hypersensitivity is mediated by which of the following immunoglobulins:

1. IgA
2. IgG
3. IgM
4. IgE

Ans. (4). IgE *(Ananthnarayan 6th ed., P. 150, Chandrasoma Taylor 2nd ed., P. 103).*

Type-I Hypersensitivity (IgE) includes:

***Local*:** Eczema, Hay fever, Asthma (Atopy)

***Systemic*:** Anaphylaxis

Examples based on type I H.S.

- Theobaldsmith phenomenon.This is anaphylaxis in guinea pigs.
- PK reaction (Prusnitz Kunster) demonstrate that IgE is homocytotropic i.e. species specific.
- Casoni's test: Immediate type (IgE) H.S.

Type-II Hypersensitivity (IgG & IgM) cytotoxic, complement mediated lysis.

Include:

a. Complement mediated lysis
b. Antibody dependent cell mediated toxicity (formerly classified as type VI)
c. Change in cellular function (former type-V)

   Increased function: Grave's disease
   Decreased function: M. Gravis

d. Phagocytosis

Examples include:

- Those with Ag on RBC

- Blood transfusion reaction
- Hemolytic anemia e.g. with IM and mycoplasma
- Those with Ag on neutrophils: Agranulocytosis
- Those with Ag on platelets: e.g. ITP
- Those with Ag on basement membrane; Goodpasture's

Type III (Immune Complex) (IgM & IgG):

Local: Arthus reaction

Systemic: Serum sickness

Examples include:

- Shick's test.
- Past streptococcal G.N.
- Detected by (Raj) Assay
- Erythema Nodosum leprosum

Type-IV (Delayed hypersensitivity):

- Cellular immunity

Examples include:

- Tuberculin test
- Lepromin test
- Contact dermatitis
- Jones-Mote Reaction (Cutaneous basophillic hypersensitivity)
- Graft rejection (Chronic)

Q.34. Virus mediated transfer of host DNA from one cell to another is known as:

1. Transduction
2. Transformation
3. Transcription
4. Integration

Ans. (1). Transduction *(Ananthnarayan 6th ed., P. 53).*

Transduction: Transfer of a portion of DNA from one bacterium in the another by means of a bacteriophage.

- Fragment from other.
- This has been proposed as a method of genetic engineering and in treatment of some inborne errors or metabolism.

Transformation: This is the transfer of genetic material through the agency of free DNA.

- May involve taking up of soluble DNA
- With host DNA and codes new species through the cell wall.
- This has been studied mainly in BPH - Bacillus, Haemophilus and Pneumococcus.

Transcription: Process by which a base sequence of mRNA is synthesized on a template of complementary DNA.

Integration: Assimilation of genetic material from one bacterium (donor) into the chromosome of another (Recipient).

Q.35. All of the following organisms are known to survive intracellularly except:

1. Neisseria meningitides
2. Salmonella typhi
3. Streptococcus pyogenes
4. Legionella pneumophila

Ans. (3).*Streptococcus pyogenes (Harrison 15th ed., P. 928, 945, 970).*

***N. meningitis*:** Meningococci that colonize the upper respiratory tract are internalized by noncilliated mucosal cell and may transverse them to enter the submucosa.

(Harrison P. 928)

***Salmonella typhi*:** Salmonellae also enter normally nonphagocytic epithelial cells by a process known as bacteria mediated endocytosis.

(Harrison P. 970)

***Legionella*:** Cell mediated immunity is the primary mechanism of host defence against legionella as it is against other intracellular pathogens.

***Streptococcus pyogenes*:** Elaborates many exotoxins which help in destroying cells.

S. pyogenes is not an intracellular bacteria.

Q.36. It is true regarding the normal microbial flora present on the skin and mucous membranes that:

1. It cannot be eradicated by antimicrobial agents.
2. It is absent in stomach due to the acidic PH.
3. It establishes in the body only after the neonatal period.
4. The flora in the small bronchi is similar to that of the trachea.

Ans. (2). It is absent in stomach due to the acidic PH *(Ananthnarayan 6th ed., P. 556).*

1. Option is wrong as normal microbial flora can be eradicated by antimicrobial agents.
2. Due to low PH of stomach it is sterile except soon after eating.
3. The mouth of infant is not sterile at birth. It contain same type of organisms as those present in mother's vagina. A healthy foetus in utero is free from microorganisms. So the flora is present in infant at birth.
4. In pharynx and trachea, flora similar to that of mouth is present. Smaller bronchi and alveoli are normally sterile.

So option 2 is correct.

Q.37. Hyperplasia with regard to tissue growth refers to:

1. An increase in the number of cells.
2. An increase in the size of cells.
3. Cellular maturation
4. Cellular differentiation from stem cells.

Ans. (1). An increase in the number of cells *(Robbins 7th ed., P. 6).*

Hyperplasia: is an increase in the number of cells in an organ of tissue, usually resulting in increased volume of the organ or tissue.

- Hyperplasia takes place if the cellular population is capable of synthesizing DNA, thus permitting mitotic division.
- Hyperplasia can be physiologic or pathologic.

1. ***Physiologic hyperplasia:*** Physiologic hyperplasia can be divided into–
   A. *Hormonal hyperplasia:* which increase the functional capacity of a tissue when needed e.g. proliferation of the glandular epithelium of the female breast at puberty and during pregnancy and in the pregnant uterus.
   B. *Compensatory hyperplasia:* which increase tissue mass after damage or partial resection e.g. capacity of the liver to degenerate, after unilateral nephrectomy, when the remaining kidney undergoes compensatory hyperplasia.
2. ***Pathologic hyperplasia:*** Most forms of pathologic hyperplasia are caused by excessive hormonal stimulation or growth factors acting on

target cells. Endometrial hyperplasia is an example of abnormal hormone induced hyperplasia. Benign prostatic hyperplasia is another common example of pathologic hyperplasia induced by response to hormones.

Q.38. All of the following statements are true regarding reversible cell injury, except:

1. Formation of amorphous densities in the mitochondrial matrix.
2. Diminished generation of adenosine triphosphate (ATP)
3. Formation of blebs in the plasma membrane.
4. Detachment of ribosome from the granular endoplasmic reticulam.

Ans. (1). Formation of amorphous densities in the mitochondrial matrix *(Robbins 7th ed., P. 24).*

Reversible cell injury:

Stems out from the widespread effects of depletion of ATP which occurs as a result of hypoxia.

***Features of reversible injury include*:**

- Cellular swelling
- Loss of microvilli
- Blebs formation
- ER Swelling: detachment of Ribosomes
- Myelin figures
- Nuclear clumping of nuclear chromatin

Irreversible injury:

Membrane damage is a central factor in pathogenesis of irreversible injury

***Feature of irreversible injury include*:**

- *Severe swelling of mitochondria:* Large, flocculant, amorphous densities develop in mitochondrial matrix (increased Ca influx).
- *Severe swelling of Lysosome:* injury to lysosomal membrane follows:

Various enzymes are released leading to:

1. Decreased basophillia
2. Nuclear changes - (i) Pyknosis, (ii) Karyolysis, (iii) Karryorrhexis
3. Protein digestion
4. Severe damage to plasma membrane.

Q.39. Barr body is found in the following phase of the cell cycle:

1. Interphase
2. Metaphase
3. G_1 Phase
4. Telophase

Ans. (1). Interphase *(Robbins 7th ed., P. 178).*

Lyon outlined the X inactivation commonly known as Lyon hypothesis. It states that only one of the X chromosome is generally active, the other X of either maternal or paternal origin undergoes heteropyknosis and is rendered inactive. Inactivation of either the maternal or paternal X occurs at random among all the cells of the blastocyst on or about the 16th day of the embryonic life and inactivation of some X chromosome persists in all the cell derived from each precursor cells. The inactive X can be seen in the interphase nucleus as a darkly staining small mass in contact with the nuclear membrane known as Barr body or X chromatin.

(Robbins 7th ed.)

More about Barr body:

Barr body also known as sex chromatin, X chromatin and drum tick. Barr body is partial inactivation and development of facultative heterochromatin in one of the two X chromosome in the interphase nuclei (Lyon 1962). It is observable after staining with orcein. Barr body occur in 20-25% cells of oral mucosa, 10% in neutrophil leucocytes, 85% in nervous tissue, 96% in amniotic fluid and chorionic epithelium of females. Any of the two

X chromosome can become heterochromatic. It begins in the late blastocyst stage (roughly 16th day of embryonic life) with germ cell develop inactivation towards the last. The X chromosome is reactivated in meiotic phase. Barr body is found in contact with nuclear envelope in oral mucosa anywhere in nucleus of nerve cells and as drumstick or small rod at one side of nucleus in neutrophils. Number of barr body is one less than the total X chromosome, one in XX (normal female), two in XXX sex complement, absent in normal human males and one in males with Klinefelter syndrome. XIST is the gene required for inactivation of X chromosome.

Q.40. Cellular and flegellar movement is carried out by all of the following except:

1. Intermediate filaments
2. Actin
3. Tubulin
4. Myosin

Ans. (4). Myosin *(Robbins 7th ed., P. 34, Gonong 20th ed., P. 12).*

Protein Subunits in Cyhtoskeleta Filaments

Protein subunits	MW	Expression	Function
Microfilaments			
Actin	42,000	Fungi, plant, animal	Structural support, motility
MreB	36,000	Rod-shaped bacteria	Width control
Microtubules			
Tubulin (a and b)	58,000	Fungi, plant, animal	Structural support, motility, cell polarity
FtsZ	58,000	Bacteria	Cell division
Intermediate Filaments			
Lamins	Various	Plant, animal	Support for nuclear membrane
Desmin, keratin, vimentin, others	Various	Animal	Cell adhesion
Other			
MSP	50,000	Nematode sperm	Motility

- **Thin filaments:** Thin filaments are composed of actin, myosin, and their associated regulatory proteins. Functioning thin filaments are essential for various stages of leukocyte movement or the ability of such cells to perform phagocytosis adequately. Some drugs and toxins target actin filaments and thus affect these processes. For example, cytochalasin B prevents polymerization of actin filaments, and phalloidin, a toxin of the mushroom Amanita phalloides, also binds actin filaments.

- **Microtubules:** Defects in the organization of microtubules can inhibit sperm motility, causing male sterility, and can immobilize the cilia of respiratory epithelium, causing interference with the ability of this epithelium to clear inhaled bacteria, leading to bronchiectasis (Kartagener's syndrome, or the immobile cilia syndrome.
- Microtubules, like microfilaments, are essential for leukocyte migration and phagocytosis. Drugs such as colchicine bind to tubulin and prevent the assembly of microtubules. Microtubules are an essential component of the mitotic spindle, which is required for cell division. Drugs that bind to microtubules (e.g., vinca alkaloids) can be antiproliferative and therefore act as antitumor agents.
- **Intermediate filaments:** These components provide a flexible intracelluar scaffold that organizes the cytoplasm and resists forces applied to the cell. Mutations in intermediate filament genes cause multiple human disorders including myopathies, neurologic disease and skin disease.

(Robbins 7th ed.)

Q.41. All of the following vascular changes are observed in acute inflammation, except:

1. Vasodialation
2. Stasis of blood
3. Increased vascular permeability
4. Decreased hydrostatic pressure

Ans. (4). Decreased hydrostatic pressure *(Robbins 7th ed., P. 49, 50)*.

Acute inflammation has three major components:

1. Alternation in vascular caliber that lead to an increase in blood flow
2. Structural change in microvascular that permit plasma proteins and leukocyte from the microcirculation.
3. Emigration of the leukocytes from the microcirculation.

Change in vascular flow and caliber:

- Vasodialation is one of the earliest manifestations of acute inflammation It follows a transient constriction of arterioles. Vasodialation first involve the arterioles and then resulting in opening of new capillary bed in the area. Thus comes about increased blood flow, which is the cause of the heat and the redness.
- Vasodialation is quickly followed by increased permeability of the microvasculature.
- The loss of fluid result in concentration of red cells in small vessels and increased viscocity of blood, reflected by the presence of dialated small vessels packed with red cells and slower blood flow, a condition termed stasis.
- As stasis develops leukocytes, principally neu-

trophils, accumulate along the vascular endothelium.

- The loss of protein from the plasma reduces the intravascular osmotic pressure and increase the osmotic pressure of the interstitial fluid. Together with the increased hydrostatic pressure owing to increased blood flow through the dialated vessels.

Q.42. Hodgkin's disease is diagnosed by finding which cells in the biopsy from lymph gland:

1. Racquet cell
2. Tzank cell
3. Reed sternberg cell
4. Lacunar cell

Ans. (3).Reed sternberg cell *(Robbins 7th ed., P. 688).*

Hodgkin lymphoma:

Lymph node involvement by the mixed cellularity type takes the form of diffuse effacement by a heterogenous cellular infiltrate which include small lymphocyte eosinophils, plasma cells and benign macrophage admixed with the neoplastic cells. Diagnostic Reed Sternberg cells and mononuclear variants are usually plentiful. In lymph node Reed Sternberg cell make the diagnosis.

Q.43. One of the following is not pencillinase susceptible:

1. Amoxicilin
2. Penicillin G
3. Piperacillin
4. Cloxacillin

Ans. (4). Cloxacillin *(K.D. Tripathi, 5th ed., P. 658).*

Classification:

1. Acid resistant alternative to penicillin G - Phenoxymethyl penicillin (Penicillin V).
2. Penicillinase resistant penicillins - methicillin, oxacillin, cloxacillin.
3. Extended spectrum penicillins:
   (a) Aminopenicillins - Ampicillin, Bacampicilin, Amoxicillin
   (b) Carboxypenicillins - Carbenicillin, Carbenicillin indanyl, Carbenicillin phenyl (Carfenicillin), Ticarcillin
   (c) Ureidopenicilins - Piperacillin, Mezlocillin.
   (d) Mecillinam (Amdinocillin)

ß lactamase inhibitors - Clavulanic acid sulbactam.

Cloxacillin: It has an isoxazolyl side chain and is highly penicillinase as well as acid resistant. It is less active against PnG sensitive organisms. Should not be used as its substitute. It is more active than methicillin against penicillinase producing staph, but not against MRSA.

Cloxacillin is incompletely but dependably absorbed from oral route, specially if taken in empty stomach. It is >90% plasma protein bound. Elimination occurs primarily by kidney, also party by liver. Plasma t1/2 is about 1 hr.

Dose: 0.25-0.5 gm orally every 6 hrs, for severe infections 0.25-1 gm may be injected i.m. or i.v. - higher blood levels are produced.

Q.44. All of the following are topically used sulphonamides except:

1. Sulphacetamide
2. Sulphadiazine
3. Silver sulphadiazine
4. Mafenide

Ans. (2). Sulphadiazine *(K.D. Tripathi, 5th ed., P. 643).*

Sulfonamides:

1. ***Sulfadiazine:*** Rapidly absorbed orally and rapidly excreted in urine. 50% plasma protein found and 20-40% acetylated. Good penetrability in brain and CSF-was is the preferred compound for meningitis.

Dose - 0.5 g QID to 2 g TDS sulfadiazine 0.5 g tab.

2. ***Sulfamethaxazole:*** Slower oral absorption and urinary excretion. A high fraction is acetylated - which is relatively insoluble - crystalluria can occur.

Dose - 1 gm BD for 2 days, then 0.5 gm BD.

Gantonol 0.5 g tab.

3. ***Sulfamoxole:*** is used when a sulfoamide alone has to be used for respiratory and urinary tract infection.

Dose - 1 g BD on first day, then 0.5 gm BD Sulfuno 0.5 g tab.

4. ***Sulfadoxine, Sulfamethopyrazine:*** They are ultralong acting compounds, action lasting >1 week because of high plasma protein binding and slow renal excretion. Because they have

caused serious cutaneous reactions large scale use of combination for prophylaxis of malaria is not recommended.

5. ***Sulfacetamide Sod:*** Highly soluble compound yielding neutral solution which is only mildly irritating to the eye in conc. upto 30%. It is used topically for ocular infection due to susceptible bacteria and chlamydia including ophthalmia neonatorum caused by ch. oculogenitalis. Locula, Albucid 10%, 20%, 30% eye drops, 6% eye ointment.
6. ***Sulfasalazine:*** used in ulcerative colitis and rheumatoid arthritis.
7. ***Mafenide:*** It is used only topically. It is active in presence of pus and against pseudomonas, clostridia sulfamylon 1% cream for surface application.
8. ***Silver sulfadiazine:*** used topically as 1% cream. Silvirin 1% cream, Argenex 1% cream with chlorhexidine (0.2%).

Q.45. A patient with grand mal epilepsy would likely be under treatment with:

1. Meprobamate
2. Pentobarbital
3. Trimethadone
4. Phenytoin

Ans. (4). Phenytoin *(K.D. Tripathi, P. 373, 378).*

Choice of antiseizures drugs

Type of Seizure	First choice drugs	Second choice drugs
1. Generalised tonic-clonic/simple partial with or without generalization	Carbamazepine, Phenytoin	Valproate, Phenobarbitone, Primidone
2. Complex partial with or without generalization	Carbamazepine, Valproate, Phenytoin	Gabapentin, Lamotrigine
3. Absence	Valproate, Ethosuximide	Clonazepam, Lamotrigine
4. Myoclonic	Valproate	Clonazepam, Lamotrigine
5. Atonic	Valproate	Clonazepam, Lamotrigine
6. Febrile seizures	Diazepam (rectal)	—
7. Status epilepticus	Diazepam (i.v.) Clonazepam (i.v.)	Phenytoin (i.v.) Phenobarbitone (i.v., i.m.)

Generalised tonic-clonic seizure is also named as GTC, Grand mal, major epilepsy.

Use of Phenytoin: Phenytoin is used for:

1. Generalised tonic - clonic, simple and complex partial seizure
2. Status epilepticus
3. Trigeminal neuralgia
4. Cardiac arrythmias

Q.46. Prolonged administration of streptomycin may result in damage to the:

1. Optic nerve
2. Facial nerve
3. Auditory nerve
4. Trigeminal nerve

Ans. (3). Auditory nerve *(K.D. Tripathi, 5th ed., P. 680, 681).*

Adverse effect of Streptomycin: About 1/5 patients given streptomycin IBD im experience vestibular disturbance. Auditory disturbance are less common.

Aminoglycosides produce toxic effect which are common to all members, but the relative propensity differs.

1. ***Cochlear damage:*** auditory nerve fibres degenerate in retrograde manner - deafness is permanent. Older patients and those with preexisting hearing defect are more susceptible.
2. ***Vestibular damage:*** Headache is usually first to appear followed by nausea, vomiting, dizziness, nystagmus, vertigo, ataxia.
3. ***Nephotoxicity:*** It manifests as tubular damage resulting in loss of urinary concentrating power, low g.f.r. nitrogen retention, albuminuria and casts.
4. ***Neuromuscular blockade:*** All aminoglycosides reduce Ach release from the motor nerve ending: interfere with mobilization of centrally located synaptic vesicles to fuse with the terminal membrane as well as decrease the sensitivity of muscle end plates to Ach.

Q.47. Dry mouth during antidepressant therapy is caused by blockade of:

1. Muscarinic acetylcholine receptors
2. Serotonergic receptors
3. Dopaminergic receptors
4. GABA receptors

Ans. (1). Muscarinic acetylcholine receptors *(K.D. Tripathi, 5th ed., P. 410, Niraj Ahuja, 4th ed., P. 174).*

Side effect of antidepressant:

***Anticholinergic action*:**

1. Dry mouth
2. Bad taste
3. Constipation
4. Epigastric distress
5. Urinary retention
6. Blurred vision
7. Palpitation *(K.D. Tripathi 5th ed.)*

Side effect of muscarinic cholinergic blockade:

1. Dry mouth
2. Urinary retention
3. Constipation
4. Cycloplegia
5. Mydriasis
6. Aggravation of glucoma
7. Delirium
8. Tachycardia
9. Memory impairment
10. Dizziness *(Niraj Ahuja, 4th ed.)*

Q.48. Which one of the following drugs has been shown to offer protection from gastric aspiration syndrome in a patient with symptoms of reflux?

1. Ondasetron
2. Metoclopramide
3. Sodium citrate
4. Atropine

Ans. (3). Sodium citrate *(K.D. Tripathi, 5th ed., P. 606).*

- Metoclopramide increase lower esophageal sphincter (LES) tone and promote gastric emptying.
- Proton pump inhibitor and H2 blocker inhibit acid secretion while antacids neutralize it.
- Alginate floats on gastric contents and prevents contact of esophageal mucosa with gastric acid.

Sodium citrate should be the choice as it reduce gastric acidity and prevent contact of acid with esophageal mucosa.

Q.49. The group of antibiotics which posses additional anti-inflammatory and immunomodulatory activities is:

1. Tetracyclines
2. Polypeptide antibiotics
3. Fluoroquinolone
4. Macrolides

Ans. (4). Macrolides *(K.D. Tripathi, 5th ed., P. 788).*

Tacrolimus is a macrolide:

- Tacrolimus (FK506) is immunosuppressant, chemically different from cyclosporine but having the same mechanism of action and is 100 times potent. It binds to a different cytoplasmic protein labelled "FKBP" but subsequent steps are same i.e. inhibition of helper T cell via calcineurium.
- Tacrolimus is administered orally as well as by I.V. infusion.
- It is particularly valuable in liver transplantation because its absorption is not dependent on bile.
- Because of more potent action it is also suitable for suppressing acute rejection that has set in.
- It causes less hypertension, hirsutism and gum hyperplasia than cyclosporine but is more likely to precipitate diabetes, cause neurotoxicity, alopecia and diarrhoea.

(K.D. Tripathi 5th ed.)

Q.50. The term refers to a type of fusion in which the formed teeth are joined only along the line of cementum:

1. Gemination
2. Fusion
3. Concrescence
4. Dilaceration

Ans. (3).Concrescence *(Shafer 4th ed., P. 39)*.

- Concrescence of teeth is actually a form of fusion which occur after root completion has been completed.
- Teeth are united by cementum only.
- It is thought to arise as a result of traumatic injury or crowding of teeth with resorption of the interdental bone so that the two roots are in approximate contact and become fused by deposition of cementum between them.
- Concrescence may occur before or after the teeth have erupted.
- The diagnosis can be frequently be established by roentgenographic examination. Since with fused teeth the extraction of one may result in the extraction of the other.

Gemination: Division of a single tooth germ by an invagination with resultatnt incomplete formation of two teeth.

Fusion: Union of two normally seprated tooth germs.

Twinning: Production of equivalent structures by division resulting in one normal and one supernumerary tooth.

Dilaceration: Angulation or bend or curve in the root or crown of formed tooth.

Q.51. Pierre Robin syndrome is associated with:

1. Micrognathia
2. Cleft of lip and palate
3. Teratology of Fallot
4. Syndactally

Ans. (1). Micrognathia *(Shafer 4th ed., P. 682).*

- Pierre Robin syndrome or Robin anomalad consist of cleft palate, micrognathia and glossoptosis.
- In this syndrome primary defect lies in arrested development and ensuing hypoplasia of the mandible, ultimately producing the characteristic "bird facies". This in turn prevent the normal descent of the tongue between the palatal shelves, resulting in cleft palate. Because of this mechanism cleft lip does not occur in association with the cleft palate.
- The most important result of this jaw malformation is respiratory difficulty.,
- The failure of support of tongue musculature occurs because of the micrognathia, allowing the tongue to fall down and backward partially obstructing the epiglottis.
- Congenital heart defects, other skeletal anomalies and ocular lesions, mental retardation may be present.

Q.52. Which is a degeneration disorder characterised by atrophic change of the deeper structures (e.g. fat, muscle, cartilage and bone) involving one side of face?

1. Scleroderma
2. Parry Romberg syndrome
3. Miescher's syndrome
4. Peutz-Jeghers syndrome

Ans. (2). Parry Romberg syndrome *(Shafer 4th ed., P. 9, 10).*

Facial hemiatrophy or Parry Romberg Syndrome is a progressive atrophy of some or all of the tissue on one side of the face occasionally extending to other parts of the body.

Etiology:

1. Trophic malfunction of the cervical sympathetic nervous system.
2. Trauma, Infection, hereditary
3. Peripheral trigeminal neuritis
4. A form of localised scleroderma.

C/F: occur in the first or second decade of life as a white line furrow or mark on one side of face or brow near the midline. This initial lesion extends progressively to include atrophy of skin, subcutaneous tissue, muscle and bone resulting in facial deformity of varying degree. There may be hollowing of cheek and the eye may appear depressed in the orbit. The cartilage of the nose, ear, larynx and palpebral tarsus also may become involved. In addition contralateral. Jacksonian epilepsy, trigeminal neuralgia and changes in the eye and hair commonly occur. Affected skin become darkly pigmented. Loss of facial hair is common. There is marked predilection for involvement of left side of the face.

Oral manifestation: Hemiatrophy of lips and tongue is reported. Growth of the teeth may be affected. There is deficiency of root development and reduced growth of jaws on the affected side. Eruption of teeth on the affected side may also be retarded.

Treatment and prognosis: No specific treatment.

Q.53. In Teacher Collin's syndrome there is:

1. Upward sloping of the palpebral fissure
2. Poorly developed or absent malar bone
3. Progenia and mandibular prognathism
4. No loss of hearing

Ans. (2). Poorly developed or absent malar bone *(Shafer 4th ed., P. 681).*

C/F of Teacher Collin's Syndrome:

1. Antimongoloid palpebral fissures with a coloboma of the outer portion of the lower lid and deficiency and of the eyelashes and sometimes the upper lid.
2. Hypoplasia of facial bone especially of the malar bone and mandible.
3. Malformation of the external ear and occasionally of the middle and internal ears.
4. Macrostomia, high palate (sometimes cleft) and abnormal position and malocclusion of teeth.
5. Blind fistulas between the angles of the ears and the angles of the mouth.
6. Atypical hair growth in the form of a tongue shaped process of the hairline extending toward the cheek.
7. Facial cleft and skeletal deformities.
8. Bird like or fish like facies.

Roentgenographic features:

1. Bodies of both malar bones tend to be grossly and symmetrically under-developed.
2. Agenesis of malar bones with non fusion of the zygomatic arches as well as absence of palatine bones.

3. Cleft palate may be seen.
4. Agenesis or hypogenesis of mandible.
5. Paranasal sinus grossly underdeveloped.
6. Mastoids appear infantile and sclerotic.
7. Auditory ossicles are often absent.
8. Cochlea and vestibular apparatus may be deficient.
9. Cranial vault is normal.

Q.54. Which of the following dentition shows the highest frequency of occurrence of supernumerary teeth?

1. Maxillary deciduous dentition
2. Maxillary permanent dentition
3. Mandibular deciduous dentition
4. Mandibular permanent dentition

Ans. (2). Maxillary permanent dentition *(Shafer 4th ed., P. 47, 48).*

Supernumerary teeth develop from a third tooth bud arising from the dental lamina near the permanent tooth bud, or possibly from splitting of permanent bud itself. There appears to be a hereditary tendency for development of supernumerary teeth. Supernumerary teeth are:

1. **Mesiodens:** is the most common supernumerary tooth situated between the maxillary central incisors occur singly, paired, Caucasian population is reported to range between 0.15 and 1.0 percent, mostly in males. Mesiodens is transmitted as an autosomal dominant trait.
2. **Maxillary fourth molar:** is the second most common supernumerary tooth and is situated distal to third molar.

Other seem with some frequency are:

3. Mandibular fourth molar.
4. Maxillary paramolars - situated between 1st and 2nd or 2nd and 3rd molar.
5. Mandibular premolars.
6. Maxillary lateral incisors.
7. Mandibular central incisors
8. Maxillary premolars

- 90% of all supernumerary teeth occur in maxilla. Supernumerary teeth are more common in permanent dentition than in deciduous dentition.
- In permanent dentition, the most common supernumerary tooth is mesiodens.
- In deciduous dentition the most common supernumerary tooth is maxillary lateral incisors.
- Multiple supernumerary teeth are found in:
  – Cleidocranial dysplasia
  – Gardener syndrome
- Supernumerary tooth is due to a single pleiotropic gene and has autosomal dominant pattern of inheritance.

Q.55. What is non characteristic of Eagle's syndrome:

1. Excessive lacrimation
2. Pain during mandibular movement
3. Stabbing type pain originate in the tonsillar regions
4. When the jaw are closed the pain subsided.

Ans. (1). Excessive lacrimation *(Shafer 4th ed., P. 864; Vinod Kapoor 1st ed., P. 281).*

- Eagle's syndrome consist of either elongation of the styloid process or ossification of the stylohyoid ligament causing dysphagia, sore throat, otalgia, glossodynia, headache, vague orofacial pain or pain along the distribution of the internal or external carotid arteries. Probably the most consistent symptom is pharyngeal pain. It is common for the difficulty to arise following tonsillectomy, presumably from fibrous tissue that forms and is stretched and rubbed over the elongated styloid process.

(Shafer)

- The patient complains of pain during swallowing. There is a feeling of foreign body lodged in the ear. The pain is increased on turning the head. This elongated styloid process may cause irritation of the sympathetic nerves on the walls of the carotid artery and produce referred pain in their distribution. Treatment of eagle syndrome is surgical management. Various approaches are:

  1. Through the lateral wall of the pharynx after doing tonsillectomy.

2. The most convenient approach is through an incision placed on the anterior border of the ramus of the mandible towards the lingual side.

(Vinod Kapoor 1st ed.)

Q.56. The most common benign tumor occurring in oral cavity is:

1. Papilloma
2. Fibroma
3. Adenoma
4. Epulis

Ans. (2). Fibroma *(Shafer 4th ed., P. 137).*

This connective tissue tumour is the most common benign soft tissue neoplasm occurring in the oral cavity.

C/F: The fibroma appears an elevated lesion of normal colour with a smooth surface and a sessile or occasionally pedunclated base. It is always a well defined slow growing lesion that occurs at any age, but is most common in the 3rd, 4th, 5th decades. It most frequently originates on the gingiva, buccal mucosa, tongue, lip, palate. Because the consistency of the fibroma may be either firm and resilient or soft and spongy.

H/F: The fibroma consist of bundles of interlacing collagenous fibres interspersed with varying numbers of fibroblast or fibrocytes and small blood vessel. The surface of the lesion is covered by a layer of stratified squamous epithelium which frequently appears stretched and shows shortening and flattening of the rate pegs.

Treatment: The treatment for fibroma is conservative surgical excision.

Q.57. In which one of the following perineural invasion in head and neck cancer is most commonly seen:

1. Adenocarcinoma
2. Adenoid cystic carcinoma
3. Basal cell adenoma
4. Squamous cell carcinoma

Ans. (2). Adenoid cystic carcinoma *(Shafer 4th ed., P. 244)*

Adenoid cystic carcinoma: The salivary glands most commonly involved by this tumour are the parotid, the submaxillary, and the accessory glands in the palate and tongue. Occur most commonly during the 5th and 6th decades of life. Many of the patient exhibit clinical manifestations of a typical malignant salivary gland tumour. Early local pain, facial nerve paralysis in case of parotid tumours, fixation to deeper structures and local invasion. Some of the lesions exhibit surface ulceration.

H/F: The adenoid cystic carcinoma is composed of small, deeply staining uniform cells resembling basal cells that are commonly arranged in anastomosing cords or a duct like pattern, the central portion of which may contain a mucoid material producing the typical cribriform, "Honey comb" or swiss cheese pattern. Characteristically the stromal connective tissue become hyalinized and surround the tumor cell forming a structural pattern of cylinders.

Treatment and Prognosis: The treatment of the adenoid cystic carcinoma is chiefly surgical. Radiation alone is not recommended.

Q.58. Name the lesion which is not a radiolucent lesion of the jaws:

1. Ameloblastoma
2. Cherubism
3. Focal periapical osteopetrosis
4. Odontogenic cyst

Ans. (3). Focal periapical osteopetrosis *(Parmod John R 1st ed., P. 223-227)*

Localised Radiolucencies:

1. Focal osteoporotic bone marrow defect
2. Surgical defect
3. Stafne cyst
4. Primordial cyst
5. Lateral periodontal cyst
6. Incisive canal cyst
7. Globulomaxillary cyst
8. Median mandibular cyst
9. Residual cyst
10. Traumatic bone cyst

Multilocular radiolucencies:

1. Odontogenic keratocyst
2. Ameloblastoma
3. Central giant cell granuloma
4. Cherubism
5. Odontogenic myxoma
6. Aneurysmal bone cyst
7. Central haemangioma of bone

Radiolucencies with ill-defined border:

1. Osteomyelitis
2. Osteoradionecrosis
3. Primary intra-alveolar squamous cell carcinoma

4. Central mucoepidermoid carcinoma of jaws
5. Metastatic carcinoma
6. Langerhans cell disease (Idiopathic histiocytosis)
7. Multiple myeloma

Generalised rarefactions:

1. Hyperparathyroidism jaw lesions
2. Osteoporosis
3. Sickle cell anaemia
4. Thalassemia
5. Massive osteolysis (Phantom bone disease)

Pericoronal radiolucencies:

Without radioopaque flecks:

1. Normal follicular space
2. Osteitis with pericornitis
3. Dentigerous cyst
4. Ameloblastic fibroma

With radioopaque flecks:

1. Ameloblastic fibroodontoma
2. Adenomatoid odontogenic tumour
3. Pindborg tumour
4. Calcifying odontogenic cyst

Localised Radioopacities:

Associated with jaws:

1. Exostosis
2. Endostosis
3. Torusmandibularis
4. Toruspalatinus
5. Idiopathic osteosclerosis
6. Condensing osteitis
7. Osteoma

8. Chondrosarcoma
9. Osteogenic sarcoma
10. Foreign bodies
11. Retained roots
12. Odontoma
13. Ameloblastic odontoma
14. Garre's osteomyelitis

Not associated with the jaws:

1. Sialolith
2. Antrolith
3. Rhinolith
4. Calcified lymphnode
5. Phlebolith
6. Cysticercosis
7. Multiple milliary osteoma
8. Calcified acne scras
9. Mineralised stylohyoid ligament

Periapical radioopacities:

1. Idiopathic osteosclerosis
2. Condensing osteitis
3. Hypercementosis
4. Periapical cemental dysplasia
5. Benign cementoblastoma
6. Benign osteoblastoma
7. Central cementifying fibroma.

Generalised Radiopacities:

1. Florid osseous dysplasia
2. Fibrous dysplasia
3. Osteopetrosis
4. Paget disease
5. Generalised cortical hyperostosis

Q.59. The best laboratory test to use in the diagnosis of lupus vulgaris in the oral cavity is:

1. Bacterial smear
2. Blood studies
3. Biopsy
4. Blood chemistry

Ans. (3). Biopsy (*Shafer 4th ed., P. 344*).

The diagnosis of lupus vulgaris (Primary tuberculosis of skin) is confirmed by microscopic examination of the tissue with demonstration of the organisms in the lesion coupled with culture and animal inoculation.

(Shafer 4th ed.)

Read text below:

Primary tuberculosis of the skin or lupus vulgaris may occur in either children or adults and is a notoriously persistent disease. Most commonly found on the head and neck especially skin of nose.

Histologically:

The nodule exhibit foci of caseous necrosis surrounded by epitheloid cells, lymphocytes and occasional multinucleated giant cells.

The small soft yellowish or brownish nodule colasec to form a single lesion. On pressure with the diascope a characteristic "apple jelly" colour is seen which is pathognomic of disease.

Q.60. Deficiency of all the three components of coagulation factor VIII result in:

1. Von willebrand's disease
2. Haemophillia-A
3. Parahaemophillia
4. Haemophillia-B

Ans. (1). Von willebrand's disease *(Shafer 4th ed., P. 753, 754).*

Von willebrand's disease: is a disease characterised by the tendency to excessive bleeding in patients who have normal platelet count, normal clotting time, normal serum fibrinogen and normal prothrombin time. Only the bleeding time prolonged.

- Inherited as autosomal dominant trait.
- Classic haemophillia is caused by a deficiency of only one of the three components of factor VIII.
- Classic Von willebrand disease is caused by decrease in all three functional components of factor VIII.

C/F: Excessive bleeding either spontaneously or following even minor trauma is the chief feature of the disease.

- Spontaneous cutaneous ecchymosis occurred in 70% of the cases.
- Bleeding into the gut and severe menorrhagia are also common.

O/M: Gingival bleeding occur after brushing of teeth.

- The disease may be discovered after dental extraction because of the prolonged and excessive bleeding.

Lab. finding: Bleeding time increased, clotting time is usually normal.

- Capillary fragility is increased with a positive tourniquet test in about 50% of case.
- Clot retraction is normal.
- Poor platelet adherence is demonstrable.

Treatment: Bleeding episodes are best treated by transfusion of plasma and or antihaemophillic factor and by local control of haemostasis.

More about VW disease:

Factor VIII von willebrand factor

1. It serves two functions:
   (a) Play a critical role in platelet aggregation.
   (b) Enhances factor VIII: C activity
2. Deficiency of factor VIII: VWF produces VW disease.
3. Factor VIII - VWF is measured by functional assay (Ristocetin test) or by an immunoassay (Factor VIII: related antigen).

Q.61. Ectodermal dysplasia is:

1. Autosomal recessive
2. Autosomal dominant
3. X-linked dominant
4. X-linked recessive

Ans. (4).X-linked recessive *(Shafer 4th ed., P. 806)*

This syndrome is characterised by a congenital dysplasia of one or more ectodermal structures and their accessory appendages, manifested primarily by hypohidrosis, hypotrichosis, hypodontia. There is abnormality of skin, hair, nails, eyes, teeth, facies, sensorineural apparatus and adnexal glandular structure. It is an X linked recessive Mendelian character. Males are affected more frequently than females.

C/F: Patient exhibit a soft smooth, thin dry skin with partial or complete absence of sweat glands. Such person can not perspire and they suffer from hyperpyrexia and an inability to endure warm temperature. The sebaceous glands and hair follicle are often defective or absent. The hair of scalp and eye brows tends to be fine scanty and blond and resemble lanugo. The moustache and beard are usually normal in appearance. The bridge of nose is depressed. The supraorbital ridges and frontal fossae are pronounced and lips protuberant. Some incidence of refractory chronic anaemia in patients with hereditary ectodermal dysplasia.

Oral finding: Manifest anodontia or oligodontia, complete or partial absence of teeth in both deciduous and permanent dentitions. Teeth present are truncated or cone shaped. Alveolar process does not develop there is a reduction from the normal vertical dimension resulting in the protuberant lips. Palatal arch is frequently high. Cleft palate may be present. Salivary gland are hypoplastic. So xerostomia occur and the protuberant lip may be dry and cracked with pseudorhagades formation. There is hypoplasia of nasal and pharyngeal mucous glands which leads to chronic rhinitis and pharyngitis, sometimes with associated dysphagia and horseness.

Treatment: There is no treatment. Partial or full denture should be constructed for functional and cosmetic purpose and reconstructed periodically as the jaws continue to grow.

Q.62. Enamel hypoplasia is not a feature of:

1. Osteopetrosis
2. Down syndrome
3. Some types of Epidermolysis bullosa
4. Cleidocranial dysplasia

Ans. (4). Cleidocranial dysplasia *(Shafer 4th ed., P. 679, 684, 839, 840).*

Oral manifestation of Osteopetrosis: Medullary space of jaws are remarkably reduced in both dominant and recessive osteopetrosis. So there is a tendency for development of osteomyelitis. Fracture of jaw during tooth extraction even when the extraction is performed without undue force may also occur because of fragility of bone. Teeth are of defective quality, enamel hypoplasia, microscopic dentinal defect and arrested root development present. Teeth are prone to dental caries. Retardation of tooth eruption due to sclerosis of bone.

Oral manifestation of Down syndrome: The patient exhibit macroglossia with protrusion of tongue, fissured tongue or pebbly tongue from enlargement of papillae. They have high arched palate. The teeth are malformed enamel hypoplasia and microdontia being the most common.

Oral manifestation of Epidermolysis bullosa: Teeth are affected in some types of epidermolysis bullosa.

1. ***Epidermolysis bullosa dystrophic, Recessive:*** Oral bullae are present. Hoarseness and dysphagia may occur as a result of bullae of larynx and pharynx. Rudimentary teeth, congenitally

absent teeth, hypoplastic teeth and crown denuded of enamel present.

2. ***Junctional Epidermolysis bullosa:*** Oral bullae are frequently very extensive and because of their extreme fragility produce serious feeding problem. Similar lesion also occur in upper respiratory tract, the bronchioles and esophagus. Severe disturbance in enamel and dentin formation of deciduous teeth.

Oral manifestation of cleidocranial dysplasia: High, narrow, arch palate actual cleft palate, maxilla under developed, enlarged mandible, prolonged retention of deciduous teeth, delay in eruption of the succedaneous teeth, Roots of teeth are short and thinner, absence or paucity of cellular cementum on permanent teeth, failure of eruption, unerupted supernumerary teeth found by roentgenographic examination, most prevalent in mandibular premolar and incisor area.

Enamel hypoplasia is absent in:

1. Epidemolysis bullosa dystropic dominant.
2. Epidermolysis bullosa simple.

Q.63. Which of the following teeth is most likely to be congenitally missing:

1. Maxillary central incisor
2. Mandibular canine
3. Mandibular second premolar
4. Maxillary first premolar

Ans. (3). Mandibular second premolar *(Bhalajhi 2nd ed., P. 92; Shafer 4th ed., P. 45).*

(A). **True anodontia:** are of two types:

(i) ***Total anodontia:*** in which all teeth are missing, may involve both deciduous and permanent dentition. e.g. Hereditary ectodermal dysplasia.

(ii) ***Partial anodontia (hypodontia or oligodontia):*** may involve one or more teeth to be normal or congenital missing.

Most common teeth missing are:

1. 3rd molars
2. Maxillary lateral incisors
3. Maxillary or mandibular second premolars

(B). **Induced or false anodentia:** occurs as a result of extraction of all teeth.

(C). **Pseudoanodontia:** multiple unerupted teeth.

In deciduous teeth most common missing teeth are maxillary lateral incisor.

Missing of teeth is due to one or more point mutations in a closely linked polygenic system, most often transmitted in an autosomal dominant pattern with incomplete penetrance and variable expressivity.

(Shafer)

Commonly missing teeth are in decreasing order of frequency.

1. Third molars
2. Maxillary lateral incisors
3. Mandibular second premolars
4. Mandibular incisors
5. Maxillary second premolar

But in above given choice third molars and maxillary lateral incisor is not given so the answer would be mandibular second premolar.

Q.64. The commonest teeth involved in transposition are:

1. Maxillary central incisor and lateral incisor
2. Maxillary canine and first premolar
3. Maxillary Ist premolar and 2nd premolar
4. Maxillary canine and lateral incisor

Ans. (2). Maxillary canine and first premolar *(White and Pharoah 4th ed., P. 309).*

Transposition:

Definition: Transposition is the condition in which two teeth have exchanged positions.

C/F: The most frequently transposed teeth are the permanent canine and first premolar (more often than the lateral incisor). Second premolars infrequently lies between first and second molars. The transposition of central and lateral incisor is rare. Transposition in the primary dentition have not been reported. It can occur with hypodontia, supernumerary teeth or the persistence of a deciduous predecessor.

Radiographic feature: Radiographs reveal transposition when the teeth are not in their usual sequence in the dental arch.

Management: Transposed teeth are frequently altered prosthetically to improve function and esthetics.

Q.65. Cafe-au-lait spots are seen in:

1. Pagets disease of bone
2. Cherubism
3. Von Recklinghausen disease
4. Von Willebrand disease

Ans. (3). Von Recklinghausen disease *(Shafer 4th ed., P. 206, 694).*

Cafe-au-lait spots are seen in diseases:

1. Polyostotic fibrous dysplasia of Jeffe's type

   These spots are irregularly pigmented melanotic spots, light brown in colour.

2. Von Recklinghausen disease (Neurofibromatosis)

   Majority of patients exhibit asymmetric area of cutaneous melanin pigmentation described as Cafe-au-lait spots.

3. Peutz-Jeghers syndrome or hereditary intestinal polyposis.
4. Hypothyroidism
5. Tuberous sclerosis.

Q.66. Name the lesion where cotton wool, multifocal radiodense conglomerates is not seen usually:

1. Gardner syndrome
2. Cementoosseus dysplasia
3. Paget disease
4. Fibrous dysplasia

Ans. (1). Gardner syndrome *(Shafer 4th ed., P. 49, 99, 163, 668).*

Feature of Gardner syndrome:

Characterised by:

1. Multiple impacted supernumerary teeth and permanent teeth.
2. Multiple polyposis of the large intestine
3. Osteomas of the bone including long bones, skull and jaws.
4. Multiple epidermoid or sebaceous cysts of the skin particularly on the scalp and back.
5. Occasional occurrence of desmoid tumours
6. Have high malignant potential.
7. It is due to single pleiotropic gene and has autosomal dominant pattern of inheritance.

So cotton wool feature is not seen in Gardner syndrome.

Q.67. Hypercementosis of entire dentition is a feature of:

1. Alber schonberg disease
2. Paget disease
3. Lathyrism
4. Low grade periapical inflammation

Ans. (2). Paget disease *(Shafer 4th ed., P. 335).*

Osteitis deformans or Paget disease of bone is a generalised skeletal disease characterised by deposition of excessive amounts of secondary cementum on the roots of teeth and by the apparent disappearance of the lamina dura of the teeth as well as by other features related to bone itself. Although the bone changes are the most prominent features of the disease, generalised hypercementosis should always suggest the possibility of the presence of osteitis deformans.

Q.68. Endemic disease means that a disease:

1. Occurs clearly in excess of normal expectancy
2. Is constantly present in a given population group
3. Exhibit seasonal pattern
4. Is prevalent among animals.

Ans. (2). Is constantly present in a given population group *(Soben Peter 1st ed., P. 917).*

Endemic: It refers to the constant presence of a disease or infectious agent within a given geographic area of population groups without importation from outside.

Other terms are:

Epidemic: A level of disease that is substantially above the usual for the population or community.

Endemic: Persistence of a disease or disability within a human population at a more or less constant level.

Exotic: Disease which are imported into a country in which they do not otherwise occur.

Epizootic: An outbreak of disease in an animal population often with implication that it may also affect human population.

Enzootic: An endemic occurring in animals.

Holoendemic: A high level of infection beginning early in life and affecting most of child population, leading to a state of equilibrium such that the adult population shows evidence of the disease much less commonly than do the children.

Hyperendemic: Persistence of a disease or disability in a human population at a very high level.

Pandemic: An epidemic usually affecting a large proportion of the population occurring over a wide geographic area such as a section of a nation, the entire nation, a continent of the world.

Prosodemic: Pertaining to infectious that maintain themselves in human population by a variety of mechanism of transmission.

Sporadic: Denoting a temporal pattern of disease occurrence in which the disease occur only rarely and without regularity.

Q.69. The brushing technique recommended for patients with periodontal disease is:

1. Scrub technique
2. Sulcular technique
3. Roll technique
4. Circular technique

Ans. (2). Sulcular technique *(Soben Peter 1st ed. P. 351 and Carranza 9th ed., P. 656).*

(Soben Peter 1st ed.)

Brushing technique	Recommended for
Bass or sulcular	Periodental patient
Charter method	Healing wound after
periodontal surgery	
Modified stillman method	Gingival recession and
root exposure	
Circular fones technique	Children

Tooth brushing Method

Method	Bristle Placement	Motion	Advantages and Disadvantages
Bass Sulcular	Apically, toward gingiva into the gingival sulcus at a 45° angle to the tooth surface.	Very short back and forth vibratory; bristle ends remain in the sulcus.	Removes plaque from cervical areas and sulcus, small area covered at one time; easily learned.
Charters	Coronally, with sides of bristles half on on gingiva at 45° to the tooth surface.	Small circular with bristle ends remaining stationary	Cleans interproximal but bristles do not go into sulcus; hard to learn; excellent gingival stimulation.
Fones Circular	Perpendicular to tooth surface.	On buccal a wide circular movement to include gingiva and tooth surfaces, on lingual, a back-forth horizontal motion.	Interproximal areas not cleaned; easy to learn; possible trauma to gingiva.
Roll Modified Stillman Technique	Apically, nearly parallel to the tooth surface, then in and over tooth surfaces.	On buccal and lingual, slight inward pressure at first, then a rolling of the head to sweep bristles over the gingiva and tooth surfaces; occlusal horizontal stroke.	Does not clean sulcus area; easy to learn; requires stillman moderate dexterity; good technique gingival stimulation.
Stillman Vibratory	On buccal and lingual, apically at an oblique angle to long axis of the tooth; ends rest on gingiva and cervical portion of tooth; on occlusal, perpendicular to occlusal surface.	On buccal and lingual, slight rotatory with bristle ends stationary; on occlusal - horizontal.	Excellent gingival stimulation; bristles do not enter sulcus; interproximal area is cleaned when the occlusal surfaces are brushed; moderate dexterity required.

Q.70. Ecologic determinants of plaque depend on all except:

1. Sugar content of diet
2. Host resistance
3. Age and sex of patient
4. Status of dentition

Ans. (3). Age and sex of patient *(Damle 1st ed., P. 23; Sturdevent 3rd ed., P. 65).*

Dental caries and periodontal disease are two most common chronic disease of oral cavity. Experimental and epidemiologic studies have demonstrated that these diseases are dependent on the microorganism present in plaque. So plaque is the cause of these diseases.

Plaque deposition depends on many factors that lead to caries formation.

1. **Dietary factors:** constituents of diet, carbohydrates, proteins, fats, minerals and vitamins.
2. **Microorganism:**
   A. Acidogenic: *S. mutans*, *Actinomyces*.
   B. Aciduric: *Lactobacilli*
   C. Other microorganisms producing IgA protease
3. **Host factors:**
   A. Tooth: Morphology of teeth, developmental defects, malocclusion etc.
   B. Saliva: Quantity, viscosity, flow rate, composition, buffering capacity etc.
   C. Genetic factors
   D. Immunological factors
4. **Other factor:** Time

So ecologic determinant of plaque depend on all factors except age and sex of patient.

(Damle 1st ed.)

Multiple factors determine the characteristics of plaque. The factors that control the presence of individual species in plaque are termed ecological determinants. These are dietary sugar, host resistance, extent and nature of shelter for bacteria, host diet, oral hygiene, status of dentition, composition of oral flora.

(Sturdevent 3rd ed.)

Q.71. The term best descries a disease transmitted to man through animals

1. Communicable
2. Transmissible
3. Zoonotic
4. Vertically transmissible.

Ans. (3).Zoonotic *(Soben peter 1st ed., P. 931).*

Zoonosis: In infection of infectious disease transmissible under natural conditions from vertebrate animals to man.

Other terms:

Anthropozoonoses: Infections transmitted from man to vertebrate animals.

Amphixenoses: Infections maintained in both man and lower vertebrate animals that may be transmitted in either directions.

Zooanthroponosis: Infections transmitted from man to vertebrate animals.

Communicable: An illness due to specific infectious agent capable of being directly or indirectly transmitted from man to man, animal to animal or from environment to man or animal.

Transmissible: Capable of being transmitted from one individual or one species to another.

Q.72. IPPM fluoride implies:

1. 1 mg of fluoride in 1 liter of water
2. 1 gm of fluoride in 1 liter of water
3. 0.1 gm of fluoride in 1 liter of water
4. 1 mg of fluoride in 100 ml of water

Ans. (1).1 mg of fluoride in 1 liter of water *(Sobenpeter 1st ed., P. 175).*

1.0 ppm = 1 mg/litre

2.2 mg sodium fluoride contains 1 mg fluoride ions

Age	Fluoride ion level in Drinking water (PPM)		
	< 0.3 PPM	0.3-0.6 PPM	> 0.6 PPM
upto 6 months	None	None	None
6 months-3yrs	0.25 mg/day	None	None
3-6 yrs	0.50 mg/day	0.25 mg/day	None
6-16 yrs	1.0 mg/day	0.50 mg/day	None

Q.73. WHO defines adolescent age between:

1. 10-19 years of age
2. 10-14 years of age
3. 10-25 years of age
4. 9-14 years of age

Ans. (1).10-19 years of age *(O.P. Ghai 5th ed., P. 41, Soben peter 1st ed., P. 910).*

Adolescence period extends from the onset of puberty till the time sexual maturation is completed. The puberty begins in girls around the age of 10 years (range 8-13 years) and in boys about the age of 12 years (range 10-15 years). It may be divided into three phages viz.

- Prepubescent (F.10-12 years; M 12-14 years)
- Pubescent (F 12-14 years; M 14-16 years)
- Post pubescent (F 14-18 years; M 16-20 years).

(O.P. Ghai)

- Adolescence defined by WHO as being between the age of 10 and 19 years (Youth 15 to 24).

(Soben peter)

Q.74. The following tests are used to check the efficiency of pasteurization of milk except:

1. Phosphatase test
2. Standard plate count
3. Coliform count
4. Methylene blue reduction test

Ans. (4). Methylene blue reduction test *(Park 18th ed., P. 477)*.

Pasteurization: May be defined as the heating of milk to such temperatures and for such period of time as are required to destroy any pathogens that may be present while causing minimal changes in the composition, flavour, nutritive value. Pasteurization kills nearly 90% of the bacteria in milk, including the more heat resistant-tubercle bacilli Q fever organisms.

- It does not kill the thermoduric bacteria.
- It does not kill bacteria spores.

There are 3 methods for pasteurization.

1. ***Holdermethod:*** Milk kept at 63-66°C for 30 minutes is rapidly cooled to 5°C.
2. ***HTST method:*** Heated to 72°C for 15 sec. and then rapidly cooled to 4°C. This is now most widely used method.
3. ***UHT method:*** Milk is rapidly heated in 2 stage the second stage usually being under pressure) to 125°C for few seconds only.

Test for pasteurised milk:

1. Phosphatase test
2. Standard platelet count
3. Coliform count

Methylene blue reduction test: is an indirect method for detection of microorganisms in milk.

Q.75. What is the colour coding of bag in hospitals to dispose off human anatomical wastes such as body parts?

1. Yellow
2. Black
3. Red
4. Blue

Ans. (1). Yellow *(Park, 17th ed., P. 567).*

There are four types of bags for disposal of bio-medical waste:

Colour coding	Waste category	Treatment option
Yellow	This bag is incinerated, so no plastic goods are collected in it. This bag is used for disposal of sputum, blood, pus, cotton, bandages, human tissue, organs body parts, items contaminated with fluids and body parts.	Incineration/ deep burial
Red	For disposable plastic items such as tubes and catheters i.v. drip set (sharp objects are disposed in this bag e.g. needles, scalpels, blades, glass that may puncture the bag.	Autoclaving/ Microwave, chemical treatment
Blue/White/ Translucent	It is a puncture proof container so sharp objects are disposed off in this bag e.g. needles, syringes, scalpel, blade glass etc.	Autoclaving/ Microwave chemical treatment and destruction/ shredding
Black	For disposal of food wastes, paper, cardboard discarded, medicines (outdated and contaminated medicines) chemical and disinfectants	Disposal and secured landfill

Q.76. Which of the following is not a method of chlorination of water?

1. Perchloron
2. Ozonation
3. Chlorine gas
4. Chloramine

Ans. (2). Ozonation *(Park 18th ed., P. 528, 529).*

For disinfecting large bodies of water, chlorine is applied either as (1) Chlorine gas, (2) Chloramine, (3) Perchloron.

1. **Chlorine gas:** Chlorine gas is the first choice because it is cheap, quick in action, efficient and easy to apply. Since chloramine gas is an irritant to eyes and poisonous, a special equipment known as chlorinating equipment is required to apply chlorine gas to water supplies. Paterson chloronome is one such device for measuring, regulating and administering gaseous chlorine to water supplies.
2. **Chloramine gas:** used in some water treatment plants. Chloramine are loose compounds chlorine and ammonia. The greatest drawback of chloramine is that they have a slower action than chlorine and therefore they are not being used to any great extent in water treatment.
3. **Perchloron or high test hypochlorite (HTH):** is a calcium compound which carries 60-70% of available chlorine. Solution prepared from HTH are also used for water disinfection.

Ozonation: Ozone is a relatively unstable gas. It is a powerful oxidizing agent. It eliminates undesirable odour, taste, and colour and removes all chlorine from the water. Most importantly ozone has a strong virucidal effect.

The drawback of ozone is that after it has done its job, it decomposes and disappears. There is no residual germicidal effect. The ozone dosage required for potable water treatment varies from 0.2 to 1.5 mg per litre.

Q.77. For the treatment of case of class III dog bite all of the following are correct except:

1. Give immunoglobulins for passive immunity
2. Give ARV
3. Immediately stitch wound under antibiotic coverage
4. Immediately wash wound with soap and water.

Ans. (3). Immediately stitch wound under antibiotic coverage *(Park 18th ed., P. 218, 219)*.

- Bite wound should not be immediately sutured to prevent additional trauma which may help the virus to spread in deeper tissue.
- If suturing is necessary, it should be done 24-48 hours later applying minimum possible stitches, under the cover of anti rabies serum locally.

(Park 18th ed.)

Classification of exposures:

- Grade I (Slight risk)
  - Licks on healthy unbroken skin
  - Consumption of unboiled milk of the suspected animals
  - Scratches without oozing of blood.
- Grade II (moderate risk)
  - Licks on fresh cuts
  - Scratches with oozing of blood
  - All bites except those of head, face, palms and fingers.

– Minor wounds less than 5 in number.

- Grade III (Severe risk)
  - All bites or scratches with oozing of blood on neck, face, palms, and fingers.
  - Lacerated wounds on any part of the body.
  - Multiple wound 5 or more in number.
  - Bites from wild animals.

Post-Exposure prophylaxis:

1. ***Wound cleansing and treatment:*** The wound should be scrubbed with soap and then flushed with water. Quarternary ammonium compounds such as 1 to 4% benzalkonium chloride, 1% cetrimonium bromide or povidone iodine solutions should be utilized. Tetanus toxoid and antibiotic prophylaxis should be administered as needed.
2. ***Passive immunisation with antirabies antiserum of either equine or human origin:*** Human rabies immune globulin (RIG) is preferred because equine antiserum may cause serum sickness. The recommended dose of RIG is 20 IU/kg.
3. ***Active immunization with antirabies vaccine:*** Vaccine such as HDCV, RVA, purified chick embryo vaccine are used.

Q.78. The diagnostic power of a test to correctly exclude the disease is reflected by:

1. Sensitivity
2. Specificity
3. Positive predictivity
4. Negative predictivity

Ans. (4). Negative predictivity *(Park 18th ed., P. 117).*

Predictive value reflects the diagnostic power of the test.

Negative predictivity: The predictive value of a negative test indicates the probability that a person has not the disease. Predictive value of negative test:

TN / FN + TN × 100

Positive predictivity: Predictive value of positive test indicate the probability that a patient with a positive result has in fact the disease. Predictive value of positive test:

TP / TP + FP × 100

Sensitivity: Ability of a test to identify correctly all those who have the disease i.e. true positive.

Sensitivity = TP / TP + FN × 100

Specificity: Ability of a test to identify correctly those who do not have the disease i.e. the negatives.

Specificity = TN / FP + TN × 100

Q.79. Cholesterol level = a + b (calorie intake) + c (physical activity) + d (body mass index): is an example of:

1. Simple linear regression
2. Simple curvilinear regression
3. Multiple linear regression
4. Multiple logistic regression

Ans. (3). Multiple linear regression *(High Yield Biostatics, P. 49; NMS Biostatics, P. 70).*

Regression:

If two variables are highly correlated, it then become possible to predict the value of the dependent variable from the value of the independent variable by using regression technique. Regression analysis is the mathematical modelling to describe the effect that one or more independent variables have on a dependent variable.

Types:

1. ***linear regression:*** The value of one variable (X) is used to predict the value of the other variable (Y) by means of a simple mathematical formula. In linear regression the dependent variable (Y) depends upon a single independent variable (X).

The linear regression equation takes the form as the equation for any straight line.

$y = a + bx$ where:–

a = is a constant k/a intercept constant

b = is the regression coefficient

x = is the independent variable.

y = is the dependent variable whose value is to be found out.

2. ***Multiple linear regression:*** More than one variable is used to predict the expected value of Y.

   Y = a + b1×1 + b2×2 + bixi, where:

   a = intercept constant

   b1 = regression coefficient for independent variable X1

3. ***Non linear regression:*** Involves more complicated mathematical forms, including logarithmic functions.

Q.80. Which one of the following statements about influence of smoking on risk of coronary heart disease (CHD) is not true:

1. Influence of smoking is independent of other risk factors for CHD
2. Influence of smoking is only additive to other risk factors for CHD
3. Influence of smoking is synergistic to other risk factors for CHD
4. Influence of smoking is directly related to number of cigarettes smoked by per day.

Ans. (2). Influence of smoking is only additive to other risk factors for CHD *(Robbins 7th ed., P. 520, Park 18th ed., P. 289).*

Risk factors for Atherosclerosis

Major	***Non quantitated***
Non-modifiable	Obesity
– Increasing age	Physical inactivity
– Male gender	Stress (type A personality)
– Family history	Post menopausal estrogen deficiency
– Genetic abnormalities	High Carbohydrate intake
Potentially controllable	
– Hyperlipidemia	Alcohol
– Hypertension	Lipoprotein LP(a)
– Cigarette smoking	Hardened (trans) unsaturated fat
– Diabetes	Chlamydia pneumoniae

Cigarette smoking is a well established risk factor in men and is thought to account for the relatively recent increase in incidence and severity of atherosclerosis in women. Smoking one or more pack of cigarette per day for several years increase the death rate from CHD by upto 200%. Cessation of smoking reduces the increases risk substantially.

(Robbins 7th ed.)

Risk factors for CHD

Not modifiable	***Modifiable***
Age	Cigarette smoking
Sex	High blood pressure
Family history	Elevated serum cholesterol
Genetic factors	Diabetes
Personality	Sedentary habits
	Stress

(Park 18th ed., P. 289)

Multiple risk factor overcome more than an additive effect.

Q.81. The most reliable criteria in Gustafson's method of identification is

1. Cementum deposition
2. Transparency of root
3. Attrition
4. Root resorption

Ans. (2). Transparency of root *(Krishan Vij 1st ed., P. 71, 72, Reddy 19th ed., P. 58).*

Criteria of age Determination by Gustafson's Method/Formula

Changes	Descriptions
1. Attrition	Wearing down of incisal or occlusal surface due to mastication (appreciable macroscopically as well as microscopically).
2. Periodontics	Retraction of gum margin and loosening of tooth (appreciable macroscopically as well as microscopically).
3. Secondary Dentin	Seen within the pulp cavity, as a result of aging/as reaction to caries and peridontosis (appreciate microscopically).
4. Cementum Apposition	At and around the root of tooth (appreciate microscopically).
5. Root Resorption	Involves both cementum and dentin (appreciable microscopically).
6. Root Transparency	Best seen on ground section of tooth. Of all the criteria, transparency of root has been considered as single most important one. The two opposite sides of an extracted or naturally fallen off tooth is ground uniformly to thin it up to less than 1 mm thickness. Then its transparency is assessed and the age is estimated with the help of a regression line prepared by studying the translucency of teeth of known ages.

Gustafson's Ranking of Structural Changes in Age Determination

Changes	Ranking and Details
Attrition = A	A-0 : No attrition A-1 : Attrition lying within enamel A-2 : Attrition reaching the dentine A-3 : Attrition reaching the pulp
Periodontosis = P	P-0 : No periodontosis P-1 : Periodontosis just begun P-2 : Periodontosis along first 1/3rd of root P-3 : Periodontosis along 2/3rd of root
Secondary Dentine = S	S-0 : No deposition of secondary dentine tissue in the pulp cavity S-1 : When secondary dentine tissue starts depositing at the upper part (in case of lower jaw and reverse in case of upper jaw) of the cavity. S-2 : When about half of the pulp cavity from above is occupied by secondary and dentine tissue S-3 : When almost whole of the cavity is filled by the dentine tissue.
Cementum Apposition = C	C-0 : Normal C-1 : A layer little greater than normal C-2 : A thick layer C-3 : A heavy layer
Root Resorption = R	R-0 : No visible resorption R-1 : Resorption only on small isolated spots R-2 : Greater loss of substance R-3 : More cementum and dentine affected
Root Transparency = T	T-0 : Transparency not present T-1 : Transparency just noticeable T-2 : Transparency over apical 1/3rd of root T-3 : Transparency over apical 2/3rd of root

(Krishan Vij 1st ed.)

Q.82. The minimum age at which an individual is responsible for his criminal act is:

1. 7 years
2. 12 years
3. 16 years
4. 21 years

Ans. (1).7 years *(Reddy 19th ed. P. 68).*

- Any act which is done by a child under seven years of age is not an offence (S. 82 IPC).
- A child between seven and twelve years is presumed to be capable of committing an offence, if he attained sufficient maturity of understanding to judge the nature and consequences of his conduct on that occasion (S. 83 IPC). This maturity is presumed in a child, unless provded otherwise by the defence.
- A child under 12 years cannot give valid consent to suffer any harm which may occur from an act done in good faith and for its benefit (S. 89 IPC).
- A person above 18 years can give valid consent to suffer any harm which may result from an act not intended or not knwon to cause death or grievous hurt (S. 87 IPC).

Q.83. Transplantation of Human organ act was passed by Government of India in:

1. 1996
2. 1993
3. 1998
4. 1994

Ans. (4).1994 *(V. Subrahmanyam 22th ed., P. 724).*

- Transplanation of human organ act provide for the regulation of removal, storage and transplantation of human organ for therapeutic purpose.
- It has been called the transplanatation of human organ act 1994 and came into effect from 4th Feb. 1995.
- Other rule is punishment for unauthorised remoal or commercial dealing and removal of names of medical practioner from registration of state and medical council or imprisonment is 2-5 years and fine 10000 rupees.

Q.84. A 25 year old female presents with 2 year history of repetitive, irresistible thoughts of contamination with dirt associated with repetitive hand washing. She reports these thoughts to be her own and distressing, but is not able to overcome them along with medications. She is most likely to benefit from which of the following therapies:

1. Exposure and response prevention
2. Systemic desensitization
3. Assertiveness training
4. Sensate focusing

Ans. (1). Exposure and response prevention *(Niraj Ahuja 4th ed. P. 88, 198).*

The patient is suffering from obsessive-compulsive disorder. The obsession is of contamination with dirt, germs, body excretions and the like. The compulsion is washing of hands or the whole body, repeatedly many times a day. It usually spread onto washing of clothes, bathroom, bedroom, door knobs and personal article gradually.

The person tries to avoid contamination but is unable to, so washing becomes a ritual.

(Niraj Ahuja, 4th ed., P. 88)

The following behaviour therapy are used for these type of patient.

1. Thought stopping (and its modifications)
2. Response prevention
3. Systemic desensitization.
4. Modelling

(Niraj Ahuja, 4th ed., P. 198)

So both response prevention and systemic desensitization therapy are used for OCD patient but according to psychiatrist response prevention is the treatment used frequently in treatment of OCD and is highly effective.

Q.85. The gold standard for the diagnosis of osteoporosis:

1. Dual energy X ray absorptiometry
2. Single energy X ray absorptiometry
3. Ultrasound
4. Quantitative computed tomography

Ans. (1). Dual energy X ray absorptiometry *(Harrison 15th ed., P. 2230).*

Several non-invasive techniques are now available for estimating skeletal mass or density. These are:

1. DXA (dual energy X-ray absorptiometry)
2. SXA (single energy X-ray absorptiometry)
3. CT (Computed tomography)
4. Ultrasound

DXA: is a highly accurate X-ray technique that has become the standard for measuring bone density in most centres. Clinical determinations are usually made of lumbar spine and hip.

- Portable DXA machines measures the heel (Calcaneus) forearm (radius and ulna) or finger (phalanges)
- DXA can also be used for measure body composition.
- In DXA technique the two X ray energies are used to estimate the area of mineralized tissue and the mineral content is divided by the area which partially corrects for body size.
- DXA is a two dimensional scanning technique and cannot estimate the depths or posteroanterior length of the bone.

Q.86. All of the following can cause osteoporosis except:

1. Hyperparathyroidism
2. Steroid use
3. Fluorosis
4. Thyrotoxicosis

Ans. (3). Fluorosis *(Harrison 15th ed., P. 2229).*

Causes of osteoporosis:

***Endocrine*:**

– Cushing's syndrome
– Thyrotoxicosis
– Hyperparathyroidism
– Acromegaly
– Adrenal insufficiency

***Rheumatological disorders*:**

– Rheumatoid arthritis
– Ankylosing spondylitis

***Hematological*:**

– Multiple myeloma
– Lymphoma
– Leukemia
– Hemophillia
– Thalassemia

***Selected inherited disorders*:**

– Osteogenesis imperfecta
– Marfan syndrome
– Homocystinuria
– Ehlers Danlos Syndrome
– Hypophosphatasia

***Drugs causing osteoporosis*:**

– Cyclosporine

- Excessive alcohol
- Glucocorticoids
- Anticonvulsants
- Aluminium
- Heparin (Chronic heparin therapy)
- Lithium

***Hypogonadal states*:**

- Turner syndrome
- Klinefelter syndrome
- Anorexia nervosa

***Other disorder*:**

- Sarcoidosis
- Multiple sclerosis
- Amyloidosis
- Immobilization

Q.87. In patients infected with HIV will have:

1. Elevated blastogenesis
2. Depressed serum globulin levels
3. High T4-T8 ratio
4. Thrombocytopenia

Ans. (4). Thrombocytopenia. *(Harrison 15th ed., P. 1889, Robbins 7th ed., P. 252, 652).*

Thrombocytopenia may be an early consequence of HIV infection. Approx 3% of patient with untreated HIV infection and CD4 + T Cell counts ≥400/μl have platelet count <15000/μl. For untreated patient with CD4 + T Cell counts <400/μl, this incidence increase to 10%.

(Harrison 15th ed.)

Major abnormalities of immune function in AIDS:

Lymphopenia:

Predominantly due to selective loss of the CD4+ helper-inducer cell subset, inversion of CD4:CD8 ratio.

Decreased T cell function in vitro:

- Preferential loss of memory T cells
- Susceptibility to opportunistic infections.
- Susceptibility to neoplasms.
- Decreased delayed type hypersensitivity.

Altered T-cell function in vitro:

- Decreased proliferative response to mitogens, allo-antigens and soluble antigens.
- Decreased specific cytotoxicity.
- Decreased helper function for pokeweed

mitogen induced B cell immunoglobulin production
- Decreased IL-2 and TFN-r production.

Polyclonal ß cell activation:

- Hypergammaglobulinemia and circulating immune complex.
- Inability to mount de novo antibody response to a new antigen or vaccine.
- Refractoriness to the normal signals for B cell activation in vitro.
- Altered monocyte or macrophage function
- Decreased chemotaxis and phagocytosis
- Decreased HLA class II antigen expression
- Diminished capacity to present antigen to T cells.
- Increased spontaneous secretion of IL-I, TNF, IL-6.

(Robbins 7th ed., P. 252)

HIV-associated Thrombocytopenia:

Thrombocytopenia is perhaps the most common haematological manifestation of HIV infection. Both impaired production and increased destruction are responsible. Infected megakaryocytes are prone to apoptosis and are impaired in terms of platelet production.

(Robbins 7th ed., P. 652)

Q.88. 5'-nucleotidase activity is increased in:

1. Bone disease
2. Prostate cancer
3. Chronic renal failure
4. Cholestatic disorder

Ans. (4). Cholestatic disorder *(Harrison 15th ed., P. 1713).*

- The activities of three enzymes - alkaline phosphatase, 5-nucleotidase, gamma glutamyl transpeptidase (GGT) - are usually elevated in cholestasis.
- Alkaline phosphatase and 5 nucleotidase are found in or near the bile canalicular membrane of hepatocytes.
- GGT is located in the endoplasmic reticulum and in the bile duct epithelial cells. Reflecting its more diffuse localization in the liver, GGT elevation in serum is less specific for cholestasis than are elevations of alkaline phosphatase or 5-nucleotidase.
- Some have advocated the use of GGT to identify patients with occult alcohol use. Its lack of specificity makes its use in this setting questionable.

Q.89. A bacterial disease that has been associated with the 3 "Rs" i.e. Rats, Rice fields and Rainfall is:

1. Leptospirosis
2. Plague
3. Meliodiosis
4. Rodent-bite fever

Ans. (1). Leptospirosis *(Harrison 15th ed., P. 1055, 1056)*.

- Leptospires are spirochetes belonging to order spirochaetales and the family leptospiraceae.
- Rodents especially rats are the most important reservoir.
- Transmission of leptospires may follow direct contact with urine, blood or tissue from an infected animal or exposure to a contaminated environment.
- Water is an important vehicle in their transmission.
- Leptospirosis occurs most commonly in tropics because the climate as well as the sometimes poor working and hygienic condition favour pathogen's survival.
- Certain occupational groups are at especially high risk included are veterinarians, agricultural workers, sewage workers, slaughter house employee and worker in the finishing industry. Such individual may acquire leptospirosis through direct exposure to or contact with contaminated water and soil.
- Most cases occur in men, with a peak incidence during the summer and fall in western countries and during the rainy season in the tropics.

Q.90. In jaundice, when there is an unconjugated hyperbilirubinemia is most likely due to:

1. Hepatitis
2. Cirrhosis
3. Obstruction of bile canaliculi
4. Increased breakdown of red cells.

Ans. (4). Increased breakdown of red cells *(Harrison 15th ed., P. 259, Robbins 7th ed., P. 887).*

Jaundice can be divided into 3 types on the basis of etiology:–

Prehepatic Jaundice:

- The cause of jaundice is increased production of bilirubin.
- For example - all causes which lead to increased hemolysis of RBCs i.e.
  - – Hereditary spherocytosis
  - – Sickle cell anemia
  - – Thallassemia
  - – Malaria
  - – Drugs such as Methyl dopa, quinine etc.
- This would lead to an unconjugated hyperbilirubinemia

Hepatic Jaundice:

- Here the cause lies within the hepatocytes
  - – either a defect in the conjugated process or
  - – in the excretion of conjugated bilirubin into the bile
- For example - all causes of hepatitis whether infection, alcohol, drugs, toxins or autoimmune – congenital hyperbilirubinemias

Post Hepatic jaundice:

- Here the cause is the obstruction of the excretion of bile into the intestines.
- For example:
  - stone in CBD
  - carcinoma in bile duct
  - pancreatic cancer etc. *(Harrison 15th ed.)*

Causes of Jaundice:

- Predominantly Unconjugated Hyperbilirubinemia
- Excess production of bilirubin
- Hemolytic anemias
- Resorption of blood from internal hemorrhage (e.g., alimentary tract bleeding, hematomas)
- Ineffective erythropoiesis syndromes (e.g., pernicious anemia, thalassemia)
- Reduced hepatic uptake
- Drug interference with membrane carrier systems
- Some cases of Gilbert syndrome
- Impaired bilirubin conjugation
- Physiologic jaundice of the newborn (decreased UGT1A1 activity, decreased excretion)
- Breast milk jaundice (ß-glucuronidases in milk)
- Genetic deficiency of UGT1A1 activity (Crigler-Najjar syndrome types I and II)
- Gilbert syndrome (mixed etiologies)
- Diffuse hepatocellular disease (e.g., viral or drug-induced hepatitis, cirrhosis)
- Predominantly conjugated hyperbilirubinemia
- Deficiency of canalicular membrane transporters (Dubin-Johnson syndrome, Rotor syndrome).
- Impaired bile flow

(Robbins 7th ed.)

Q.91. Hypercalcemia associated with malignancy is most often mediated by:

1. Parathyroid hormone (PTH)
2. Parathyroid hormone related protein (PTHrP)
3. Interleukin-6 (IL-6)
4. Calcitonin

Ans. (2). Parathyroid hormone related protein (PTHrP) *(Harrison 15th ed., P. 632).*

Hypercalcemia of malignancy: Hypercalcemia of malignancy, the most common paraneoplastic endocrine syndrome is responsible for approximately 40% of all hypercalcemia. Two type occur

1. ***Humoral hypercalcemia of malignancy (40%):*** caused by circulating hormones.
2. ***Local osteolytic hypercalcemia (LOH):*** caused by local paracrine factors secreted by cancer within bone.

Parathyroid-related peptide (PTHrP) cause nearly all cases of HNM while the mediators of LOH in bone are heterogeneous.

Pathogenesis: 80% of patients with hypercalcemia malignancy have HNM. PTHrP is composed of 139 to 173 aminoacids. PTHrP is detected in plasma in 80% of cancer patient with hypercalcemia. 20% of patients with hypercalcemia have LOH in which hypercalcemia is caused by local production of hormone or cytokines by cancers that have spread to bone or bone marrow.

Clinical manifestation: The initial symptoms and sign of hypercalcemia (Ca level $\geq$2.6 mmol/L) include malaise, fatigue, confusion, anorexia, bone pain, polyuria, polydipsia, weakness, constipation, nausea, vomiting, neurologic symptoms are confusion, lethargy, coma, death.

Common Paraneoplastic Endocrine Syndromes

Syndrome	Proteins	Tumors Typically Associated with syndrome
Hypercalcemia of malignancy	Parathyroid hormone-related peptide (PTHrP) Parathyroid hormone (PTH)	Non-small cell lung cancer • Breast cancer • Renal cell carcinoma • Head and neck cancer • Bladder cancer • Myeloma
Syndrome of inappropriate • Antidiuretic hormone • Secretion (SIADH)	Arginine vasopressin (AVP) Atrial natriuretic peptide	• Small cell lung cancer • Head and neck cancer • Non-small cell lung cancer
Cushing's syndrome	Adrenocorticotropic hormone (ACTH) Corticotropin-releasing hormone (CRH)	• Small cell lung cancer • Carcinoid tumors
Acromegaly	Growth hormone - releasing hormone (GHRH), Growth hormone (GH)	• Carcinoid tumors • Small cell lung cancer • Pancreatic islet cell tumors
Gynecomastia	Human chorionic gonadotropin (hCG)	• Testicular cancer • Lung cancer • Carcinoid tumors of the lung and gastrointestinal tract
Non-islet cell tumor hypoglycemia	Insulin-like growth factor-2 (IGF-2)	• Sarcomas

Q.92. Heme is converted to bilirubin mainly in:

1. Kidney
2. Liver
3. Spleen
4. Bone marrow

Ans. (3). Spleen *(Harrison 15th ed., P. 255).*

- Bilirubin, a tetrapyrrole pigment is a breakdown product of home. The following are source of bilirubin.
  1. 70 to 80% of the 250 to 350 mg of bilirubin produced each day is derived from the breakdown of haemoglobin in senescent red blood cells.
  2. Prematurely destroyed erythroid cells in bone marrow, and
  3. Turnover of haemoprotein such as mylo-globin and cytochrome found in tissue throughout the body.
- The formation of bilirubin occurs in reticuloendothelial cells. Primarily in the spleen and liver.

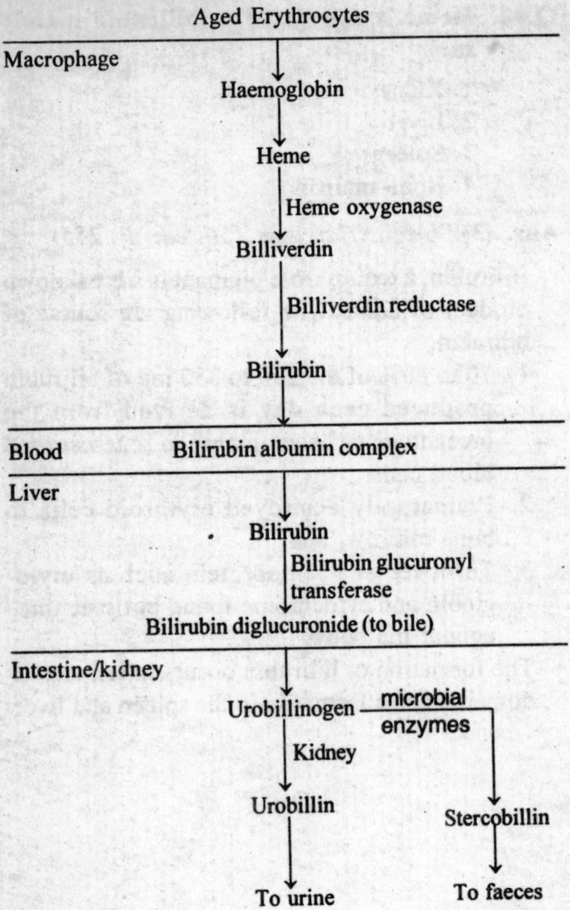
Aged Erythrocytes
Macrophage
Haemoglobin
Heme
Heme oxygenase
Billiverdin
Billiverdin reductase
Bilirubin
Blood
Bilirubin albumin complex
Liver
Bilirubin
Bilirubin glucuronyl transferase
Bilirubin diglucuronide (to bile)
Intestine/kidney
Urobillinogen
microbial enzymes
Kidney
Urobillin
Stercobillin
To urine
To faeces

Q.93. HIV can be detected and confirmed by:

1. Polymerase chain reaction (PCR)
2. Reverse Transcriptase PCR
3. Real time PCR
4. Mimic PCR

Ans. (2). Reverse Transcriptase PCR *(Harrison 15th ed., P. 1878).*

- For the detection of HIV-RNA the use of reverse-transcriptase PCR (RT-PCR) and bDNA technique is increasing.
- RT-PCR (Amplicor) and β-DNA (Quantiplex) are the two assays predominantly used in providing a diagnostic tool by measuring an monitoring levels of HIV-RNA in settings where measurements of anti-HIV antibodies may be misleading such as in acute infections and neonatal infections.
- DNA-PCR is also used for making a diagnosis of HIV infection by amplifying HIV Proviral DNA from peripheral mononuclear blood cells.
- RT-PCR is also useful for amplifying a defined areas of the HIV-genome for sequence analysis and has become an important technique for studies of sequence diversity and microbial resistance to antiretroviral agent.

Q.94. Differential expression of same gene depending on parent of origin is referred to as:

1. Genomic imprinting
2. Mosaicism
3. Anticipation
4. Non-penetrance

Ans. (1). Genomic imprinting *(Harrison 15th ed., P. 392).*

According to traditional mandelian principles, the parental origin of a mutant gene is irrelevant for expression of the phenotype. Exception-X inactivation prevents the expression of most genes on one of the two X chromosome in every cell of a female. Gene inactivation also occurs on selected regions of autosomes. This is called Genomic imprinting, leads to preferential expression of an allele depending on its parental origin.

Examples:

1. Parder willi syndrome
2. Angelman syndrome

Mosaicism refers to the presence of two or more genetically distinct cell lines in the tissue of an individual.

Examples:

MC Cune-Albright syndrome

Anticipation: In this when repeat length increase from one generation to the next, disease manifestations may worsen or be observed at an earlier age, this phenomenon is referred to as Anticipation.

Eg. Repeated sequence occur in Huntington disease, spinocerebellar ataxia, Friederich ataxia, Fragile X syndrome.

Non-penetrance: if all carriers of a mutant express the phenotype and if some of them express, then called non-penetrance or incomplete penetrance.

Eg. Hypertrophic cardiomyopathy by mutation in myosin binding protein C gene.

Q.95. In chronic arsenic poisoning the following sample can be sent for laboratory examination, except:

1. Nail clippings
2. Hair samples
3. Bone biopsy
4. Blood sample

Ans. (4). Blood sample *(Harrison 15th ed., P. 2594).*

- Arsenic is present in hair, nails, bone for long time and it is rapidly cleared from blood.
- Blood sample is useful in acute arsenic poisoning is not a reliable for diagnosis of chronic arsenic poisoning.

Read text below:

Arsenic poisoning:

- Tasteless: odourless: mixed with food, drinks, paan.
- Associated with spasm.
- Fatal dose - 120-200 mg.
- Resemble with cholera
- Treatment is by freshly precipitated hydrated ferric chloride.
- Postmortem - Rigor moritis lasts longer
- Not destroyed by heat - Stomach mucosa is red velvet.

Chronic poisoning:

C/F: Nausea, vomiting, skin rashes, hyperkeratosis

– Rain drop type pigmentation.

– Mee's line (5 weeks after exposure)

– Tingling and numbness
– Arsenic neuritis

Postmortem: Retardation of decomposition

- Arsenic deposited in hair, nails, end of long bones and can be detected even in charred remains after the body is burnt.
- Marsh test - to detect the presence of arsenic even upto 1/1000 of a mg.

Q.96. Which one of the following serum levels would help in distinguishing an acute liver disease from chronic liver disease?

1. Aminotransaminase
2. Alkaline phosphatase
3. Bilirubin
4. Albumin

Ans. (4). Albumin *(Harrison 15th ed., P. 1713).*

- Serum albumin is not a good indicator of acute or mild hepatic dysfunction. Only minimal changes in the serum albumin are seen in acute liver conditions such as viral hepatitis, drug related toxicity and obstructive jaundice.
- In hepatitis, albumin levels below 3 gm/dl should raise the possibility of chronic liver disease.
- Hypoalbuminemia is more common in chronic liver disorders such as cirrhosis and usually reflects severe liver damage and decreased albumin synthesis.

Q.97. Androphonia can be corrected by doing:

1. Type I thyroplasty
2. Type II thyroplasty
3. Type III thyroplasty
4. Type IV thyroplasty

Ans. (4). Type IV thyroplasty *(The larynx by Marvin P. Fried 2nd ed., P. 248; Dhingra 3rd ed. P. 364).*

Thyroplasty: was introduced by Isshiki to describe a series of operation in which the thyroid cartilage is surgically modified to effect changes in the voice.

Laryngeal framework surgery:

- Isshiki Type I: Medialization
- Isshiki Type II: Lateralization (Expansion thyroplasty)
- Isshiki Type III: Anterior retrusion (Retrusion thyroplasty)
- Isshiki Type IV:
  - Anterior protrusion (Cricothyroid approximation).
  - Arytenoid adduction

Type I: is the most widely used form of thyroplasty. It is probably the treatment of choice for most cases of glottic insufficiency, which is a relatively common problem and the most common indication for thyroplasty.

Indications:

1. Vocal fold paralysis or paresis
2. Immobile vocal fold for causes other than laryngeal cancer.

3. Presbylaryngis or other causes of bowed vocal folds.
4. Sulcus vocalis and related deformities.
5. Scarred or absent vocal folds e.g. postcordectomy.

Type II: Vocal fold lateralization and decreased force of glottic closure is the good of type II thyroplasty.

Indication: The main indication for Type II thyroplasty is adductor spasmodic dysphonia.

Type III: This type combines the features of expansion and retrusion thyroplasty and can be useful in treating selected cases of spasmodic dysphonia.

Indication: This thyroplasty is used mainly for adductor spasmodic dysphonia. Also used for refractory mutational falsetto and for inappropriately high pitched male voices.

Type IV: The simplest technique is cricothyroid approximation. It is used to raise vocal pitch.

Indication: The only essential indication for Type IV thyroplasty is an inappropriately low vocal pitch in the absence of treatable vocal fold pathology. Although it might be helpful in cricothyroid muscle paralysis, the most common use is in androphonia and gender reassignment (transsexual) women with residual low pitched (male) voices.

Q.98. Abbey-estlander flap is used in the reconstruction of:

1. Buccal mucosa
2. Lip
3. Tongue
4. Palate

Ans. (2). Lip *(The Surgical head and neck by Watkinson 4th ed., P. 284; Kruger 6th ed., P. 488).*

Abbe Eslander flap for angle of lip tumours:

This flap is performed to reconstruct defects that require partial commissure reconstruction. The flap is marked out rotated and sewn in, and a new commissure is formed. Care should be taken not to damage the pedicle and the only major problem with this technique is that it result in a rounded commissure which often leads to postoperative asymmetry. Full commissure reconstruction require either double rhomboid cheek flaps with vermillion advancement or free tissue transfer. Because of difficulty in creating a new commissure, every attempt should be made to retain the angle of mouth. So Abbe-Estlander flap is used to reconstruct tumours of the commissure.

Q.99. The most common and earliest manifestation of carcinoma of glottis is:

1. Hoarseness
2. Haemoptysis
3. Cervical lymphnode
4. Stridor

Ans. (1). Hoarseness *(Bhargava 6th ed., P. 301-304, Dhingra 2nd ed., P. 164).*

Carcinoma of the vocal Cords (Glottic):

It is one of the commonest types of laryngeal carcinomas.

Aetiology:

1. ***Age:*** It is usually seen after the age of 45 years sarcoma may occur at an early age.
2. ***Sex:*** It is very common in males.
3. ***Premalignant conditions:***
   (a) Single papilloma
   (b) Leucoplakia
4. ***Precipitating Factors:***
   (a) Smoking
   (b) Chronic irritation
   (c) Atmospheric pollution

<u>*Pathology:*</u> Majority of malignancies are squamous cell carcinomas. Adenocarcinomas, basal cell carcinomas or sarcomas.

Symptoms:

1. Hoarseness is the earliest symptom and prompts the patient to approach early for the medical help.
2. Cough
3. Raw sensation

4. Blood stained sputum
5. Stridor
6. Lymph nodal metastasis
7. Widening of the larynx.
8. Dysphagia

Signs:

Site: Anterior half of the vocal cord from its edge or the upper site.

Morphology: Cauliflower like growth, but it may be ulcerative, leucoplakia may undergo malignant change.

Spread:

1. Continuity
2. Lymphatic
3. Blood stream

Investigations:

1. Biopsy: Performed by direct laryngoscopy or microlaryngoscopy is diagnostic.
2. Routine investigation
3. VDRL
4. Radiograph of the chest
5. Soft tissue radiograph
6. CT Scan

Differential Diagnosis:

It is similar to that of chronic laryngitis.

Treatment: the treatment depends upon many factors.

1. Stage of the growth
2. Histopathology
3. General fitness of the patient

4. Facilities available
5. Occupation

Advanced cases: Palliative treatment is advised.

a. Analgesia for relieving pain.
b. Antibiotics for controlling infection.
c. Tracheostomy for stridor.
d. Ryle tube feeding or gastrostomy for dysphagia.
e. Chemotherapy
f. Irradiation.

Q.100. The most lethal of complications due to blood transfusion is:

1. Jaundice
2. Antigen antibody reaction
3. Hepatitis B transmission
4. HIV transmission

Ans. (2). Antigen antibody reaction *(Bailey and Love 24th ed., P. 64, 65; S. Das 3rd ed., P. 4).*

Complications of blood transfusion:

1. Congestive cardiac failure
2. Transfusion reaction
3. Infections
4. Thrombophlebitis
5. Air embolism
6. Coagulation failure

(A) **Transfusion reactions:**

1. *Incompatibility* (antigen-antibody reaction): This should be avoided if the correct procedure of grouping and cross matching have been adopted. The patient develop a rigor, fever and pain in the loins and may become extremely alarmed. The transfusion should be stopped immediately and a fresh specimen of venous blood and urine from the patient must be sent together with the residue of all the used units of donor blood to the laboratory for checking. A close watch should be kept on the patient's pulse, blood pressure, and urinary output. Frusemide 80-120 mg iv is given to provoke a diuresis and repeated if the urine output falls below 30 ml per hour. Dialysis may be necessary.

2. Simple pyrexia reactions
3. Allergic reactions
4. Sensitization to leucocytes and platelets
5. Immunological sensitisation

(B) **Infections:** Serum hepatitis, HIV, Bacterial infection, malaria.

(C) **Thrombophlebitis**
(D) **Air embolism**
(E) **Coagulation failure** — due to dilution of clotting factors/platelets, disseminated.intravascular coagulation *(Bailey and Love 24th ed.)*

If haemolysis is severe it may cause acute renal tubulernecrosis renal failure and death of individual

(S. Das 3rd ed.)

Q.101. Which of the following statement is true with reference to Glasgow Coma Scale?

1. In the first 24 hrs following a head injury an overall score of 11 indicates a good prognosis
2. An overall score of less than 9 indicates a poor prognosis.
3. Give an accurate impression of the neurological status.
4. Cannot be assessed in an unconscious patient.

Ans. (2). An overall score of less than 9 indicates a poor prognosis *(Bailey and Love, 24th ed., P. 600, 601).*

Read text below:

Glasgow coma scale (GCS). The maximum score is 15. The minimum is 3.

Eye opening	Verbal response	Best motor response
Spontaneous - 4	Oriental - 5	Obeys - 6
To speech - 3	Confused conversation-4	Localises - 5
To pain - 2	Inappropriate words-3	Withdraws - 4
Nil - 1	Incomprehensible sounds - 2	Abnormal flexion - 3
	Nil - 1	Extension response-2
		Nil - 1

- Score of less than 7 suggest coma. Score of 9 or more excludes coma. Most cases with score of 8 are also comatose.

Classification of head injury severity:

Classification	Range of Glasgow Coma Scale Score
Mild	GCS $\geq$ 13
Moderate	GCS 9 to 12
Severe	GCS < 8

- Patient with a GCS score of 8 or less and patient with lateralizing neurologic findings are at particularly high risk and should undergo head CT as soon as they are haemodynamically stable.
- Level of consciousness is most commonly assessed by the GCS score.
- The level of GCS score in an indicator of overall prognosis and also is predictive of likelihood of neurosurgical intervention.
- The GCS score is useful because it is simple and objective and can be repeated serially.
- A decrease of even 1 or 2 points in the GCS score is indicative of a significant change in neurologic status and demands prompt reevaluation and treatment.
- The GCS is heavily weighted towards higher cognitive function and the presence of acute drug or alcohol intoxication can greatly lower scores in eye opening and verbal categories, even in the absence of brain injury. Change in motor component of the GCS are most predictive of serious anatomic injury to the brain. It is impossible to have a GCS score in severe head injury range (GCS $\leq$8) without changes in the motor component.

Q.102. Lumbar sympathectomy is of value in the management of:

1. Intermittent claudication
2. Distal ischemia affecting the skin of the toes
3. Artriovenous fistula
4. Back pain

Ans. (2). Distal ischemia affecting the skin of the toes *(S. Das 4th ed., P. 154, 226, Bailey and Love 23rd ed., P. 207).*

Main indication of Lumbar Sympathectomy:

1. Rest pain and minor ulceration
2. Burger disease
3. Raynaud disease and other vasospastic condition.
4. Senile gangrene or diabetic gangrene (distal ischaemia)
5. Hyperhidrosis
6. Causalgia.
   - Intermittent claudication is managed by conservative means such as stoppage of smoking, diet, managing lipid abnormalities, exercises.
   - Sympathectomy is not very effective in claudication, but occasionally it may relieve ischaemic rest pain and ulceration.

Q.103. Hand over mouth technique was first described by:

1. Dr. Evangeline Jordan
2. Addelson and Gold fried
3. Dr. G.V. Black
4. Dr. Goldman

Ans. (1). Dr. Evangeline Jordan *(Shobha Tondon 1st ed., P. 151, Damle 1st ed., P. 19).*

Various techniques and their discover:

- Home: Dr. Evangeline Jordan (1920)
- TSD: Addleslon (1959)
- Modelling: Bandura (1969)
- Desensitization: Joseph Wolpe (1975)
- Negative reinforcement: Stokes and Kennedy (1980)
- Audio analgesia: Gardner, Licklider (1959)
- Biofeed back: Buonomono (1979)
- Coping: La Zaue (1980)
- Emotion regulating cognitions: Sandra L. Curry (1988)
- Voice Control: Henry and Marilyn (1984)
- Signal system: Musslemann (1991)
- Hypnosis: Romanson (1981)
- Hypnodontics: Richardson (1980)
- Aversive conditioning: Patricia P Hagan (1984)
- Physical restraints: Kelly (1976)

More about HOME technique: The purpose of HOME is to gain the attention of a child so that a communication can be achieved.

Indication:

1. A healthy child who can understand but who

exhibits defiance and hysterical behaviour during treatment.

2. 3-6 years old.
3. A child who can understand simple verbal commands.
4. Children displaying uncontrollable behaviour.

Contraindications:

1. Child under 3 years of age.
2. Handicapped child / immature child, frightened child
3. Physical, mental and emotional handicap.
4. Asthmatic, mouth breather.

Technique: After determining the child behaviours the dentist places his hand over child's mouth and behaviour expectations are calmly explained. The child is told that the hand will be removed as soon as appropriate behaviour begins. When the child responds the hand is removed and appropriate behaviour is reinforced.

Several variations of HOME:

1. Hand over mouth the airway unrestricted.
2. Hand over mouth and the nose and the airway restricted.
3. Towel held over mouth only.
4. Dry towel held over nose and mouth.
5. Wet towel held over nose and mouth.

Q.104. As age advances, the human profile generally:

1. Remain the same.
2. Increase in convexity.
3. Decrease in convexity.
4. Decrease in concavity.

Ans. (3). Decrease in convexity *(McDonald 7th ed., P. 636).*

- Following birth, the face increase in size to a greater extent than does calvarial size. Bell proposes that by adulthood, the ideal face should be equally proportioned in forehead, midface and lower face heights.
- Enlow has demonstrated that the facial profile flattens as the face ages. Nose and chin become more prominent and the lips less pronounced as the face ages.
- Every healthy individual, regardless of the overall craniofacial pattern experiences profile flattening and face height increase relative to cranium.
- Criteria for facial idealness is age dependent. Because face elongates and profile become less convex with maturity, ideal criteria appropriate for the adult face would not necessary apply to the younger face.

Q.105. What is the average amount of Leeway space available in upper arch?

1. 0.9 mm
2. 1.8 mm
3. 3.5 mm
4. 5.0 mm

Ans. (2).1.8 mm *(Rani 3rd ed., P. 95, Bhalajhi 2nd ed., P. 56).*

Leeway Space of Nance: The combined mesiodistal width of CDE is larger than the combined mesiodistal width of underlying 345. The difference in mesiodistal width of CDE and 345 is referred to as Leeway space of Nance. This is 1.7 mm on either side of lower arch total it amounts to 3.4 mm in lower arch. Whereas it is only 0.9 mm on either side of upper arch amounting to 1.8 mm in upper arch. This Leeway space allows the mesial movement of lower molar thereby it corrects the Flush terminal plane relationship to class I molar relationship.

Q.106. Who proposed the operant conditioning theory of child psychology?

1. Pavlov
2. Skinner
3. Jean Piaget
4. Sigmond freud

Ans. (2). Skinner *(Shobha Tondon 1st ed., P. 125, Sobenpeter 1st ed., P. 553)*

Psychodynamic theories:

1. Classical psychoanalytical theory (Psychosexual) by Sigmund Freud (1905)
2. Developmental task theory (Psychosocial) by Erik Erikson (1963).
3. Hierarchy of needs by Abraham Maslow (1954).

Behaviour learning theory:

1. Classical conditioning theory by Ivan Pavlov (1927)
2. Operant conditioning theory by B.F. Skinner (1938)
3. Social learning theory by Albert Bandura
4. Theory of cognitive development by Jean Piaget (1952).
5. Transactional Analysis theory by Eric Berne (1964).

Operant conditioning theory:

Skinner (1938)

According to this theory, the consequence of behaviour itself act as a stimulus and affect future behaviour. Since the behaviour acts upon the environment it is called and operant. Skinner described 4 types of operant conditioning.

1. Positive reinforcement
2. Negative reinforcement
3. Omission
4. Punishment

Positive and negative reinforcement are the most suitable type of operant conditioning for a dental office while the other 2 types of operant conditioning should be used with caution.

Q.107. Speech retardation may be considered if the child does not talk by:

1. 12 months
2. 18 months
3. 24 months
4. 36 months

Ans. (4).36 months *(McDonald 5th ed., P. 843, 844)*.

- Upto 24 month of age child develop language milestone. At 24 month of age the child pronounce (I, me, you and so forth inappropriately).
- Significant (9-12 months) delay in the attainment of milestones is an important indicator of potential abnormality.

Q.108. Caries activity test that gives a quantitative determination of the acidogenic microorganism in the oral cavity:

1. Fosdick test
2. Snyder test
3. Albans test
4. Blawary reductase test

Ans. (2). Snyder test *(Damle 1st ed., P. 47, 48).*

Snyder test: This test measure the ability of microorganism in saliva to form acids from carbohydrate media. 0.2 cc of saliva is pipetted into the media, which is incubated at 37°C upto a period of 72 hours. The media contains:

1. Bactopeptone - 20 gms
2. Dextrose - 20 gms
3. Sodium chloride - 5 gms
4. Agar - 16 gms
5. Bromocresol green 0.02 gms

Bromocresol green being an indicator change the colour from green to yellow in the range of PH of 5.4-3.8. The colour change is then correlated with the caries activity.

Alban test: is a modification of the snyder test. It use less agar i.e. 5 ml per tube. The saliva is drooled directly into the tube and the tubes are incubated for 4 days at 37°C. The colour change is noted from bluish green to yellow and the depth to which the change has occurred is noted.

Blawary reductase test: measures the activity of the salivary enzyme reductase. The sample is collected mixed with an indicator i.e. diazoresorcinol. The change in colour are measured after 30 sec. and 15 minutes and are taken as a measure of caries activity.

Fosdick calcium dissolution test: measure the amount of powdered enamel dissolved by acid in 4 hours, when mixed with glucose and the patients saliva. The extent of increased calcium is supposedly a direct measure of the degree of caries susceptibility. However this test is not generally suited for office proceedure.

Q.109. The threshold dose of fluoride that requires immediate emergency treatment and hospitalization in acute fluoride toxicity is:

1. 4 mg
2. 5 mg
3. 6 mg
4. 7 mg

Ans. (2).5 mg *(Damle 1st ed., P. 251).*

PTD: The probably toxic dose of fluoride is the minimum dose that could cause serious or life threatening systemic signs and symptoms and that should trigger immediate therapeutic intervention and hospitalization. The exact dose can not be accurately stated but taking into account all the reported doses which have caused complications, we can say that an oral fluoride dose of 5.0 mg/kg body weight should be considered as PTD. This does not mean that dose below 5 mg/kg body weight are harmless.

Effect	Dosage	Duration
Dental fluorosis	> 2 times optimal	until 5 year of age
Skeletal fluorosis	10-25 mg/day	10-20 years
Kidney damage (in animals)	5-10 mg/kg	6-12 months

Sign and symptoms of acute fluoride toxicity:

1. Nausea
2. Vomiting
3. Epigastric distress
4. Excess salivation

5. Diarrhoea
6. Mucus discharge from nose and mouth
7. Headache
8. Sweating
9. Barely detectable pulse
10. Hypotension
11. Cardiac arrhythmias
12. Disturbance in electrolyte balance i.e. hypocalcemia, hypokalemia
13. Respiratory and metabolic acidosis
14. Coma

Q.110. When is the first evidence of calcification of primary teeth?

1. 4 months in utero
2. 4 and 1/2 months in utero
3. 5 months in utero
4. 6 months in utero

Ans. (1).4 months in utero *(Shobha Tondon 1st ed., P. 723 Appendix).*

Hard tissue formation:

Deciduous detention:

Maxillary:

– Central incisor - 4 mo in utero
– Lateral incisor - 4½ mo in utero
– Cusped - 5 mo in utero
– First molar - 5 mo in utero
– Second molar - 6 mo in utero

Mandibular:

– Central incisor - 4½ mo in utero
– Lateral incisor - 4½ mo in utero
– Cusped - 5 mo in utero
– First molar - 5 mo in utero
– Second molar - 6 mo in utero

Permanent detention:

Maxillary:

– Central incisor - 3-4 mo
– Lateral incisor - 10-12 mo
– Cusped - 4-5 mo
– First bicuspid - $1\frac{1}{2}$ - $1\frac{3}{4}$ yrs
– Second bicuspid - 2-$2\frac{1}{4}$ yrs
– First molar - At birth

– Second molar - $2\frac{1}{2}$-3 yrs
– Third molar - 7-9 yrs

Mandibular:

– Central incisor - 3-4 mo
– Lateral incisor - 3-4 mo
– Cusped - 4-5 mo
– First bicuspid - $1\frac{3}{4}$-2 yrs
– Second bicuspid - $2\frac{1}{4}$-$2\frac{1}{2}$ yrs
– First molar - At birth
– Second molar - $2\frac{1}{2}$-3 yrs
– Third molar - 8-10 yrs

Q.111. By what age does the startle and grasp reflex disappear?

1. 1 year
2. 1½ year
3. 2 year
4. 3 year

Ans. (3).2 years *(Shobha Tondon 1st ed., P. 57, O.P. Ghai 5th ed., P. 124).*

Startle reflex: It is similar to moro reflex but is initiated by a sudden noise or any other stimulus. In this reflex, the elbows are flexed and the hands remain closed. There is less of the embrace, less outward and inward movement of the arms. Grasp reflex disappear by 24 months.

Various other reflex are:

1. ***Moro's reflex:*** Develop by 28 weeks gestation.
   Disappear by 3 months.
2. ***Tonic neck reflex:*** Appear by 2 to 3 months
   Disappear by 8 months
3. ***Palmer grasp reflex:*** Develop by 28 weeks
   Disappear by 4 months
4. ***Sucking reflex:*** Appear by 14 weeks of gestation.
5. ***Rooting reflex:*** Develops by 28 weeks of gestation.
6. ***Grasp reflex:*** Appear by 34 weeks.
   Disappear by 24 months.
7. ***Crossed extension:*** appear by 32 weeks.
8. ***Gag reflex:*** appear by 18½ weeks of IU life.
9. ***Cry:*** start as early as 21-29 weeks of IU life.
10. ***Parachute reflex:*** appear by 6-9 months.

11. ***Landau reflex:*** Present for 3 months. Disappear at 1 year of age.
12. ***Pincer grasp:*** Develop by 8th month of age

Read the reflexes in detail from the above given references.

Q.112. Mouth guards to prevent accidents to teeth are most practical for:

1. All children
2. All persons engaged in contact sports.
3. Automobile passengers
4. Persons on organized athletic team.

Ans. (4). Persons on organized athletic team *(Damle 1st ed., P. 204).*

- A mouth guard is a flexible appliance made from plastic and it is most commonly used by athletes. Incidence of traumatic injuries is most commonly seen in those who indulge in contact sports.
- Mouth guard helps prevent injuries and thus protect an individual from the dreadful consequences like concussion injuries, jaw fracture, cerebral haemorrhage etc.
- Protect dentition from several bruises and protect soft tissues of oral cavity. Children undergoing orthodontic therapy are highly benefitted by using mouth guard.

Different types of mouth guard:

1. ***Stock:*** This mouth guard has lowest cost among the available mouth guards.

Disadvantage:

- This mouth guard offer least protection
- Interfere with speech.
- Not very acceptable.

2. ***Mouth formed appliance:*** This comes as a shell liner. It is a boil and bite product. It consist of shell lined with acrylic or rubber. It is placed in the mouth and the material is moulded

to fit properly. The lining of the boil and bite mouth guard is first immersed in boiling water for about 10-20 sec and then immersed in cold water and then adapted.

This type of mouth guard is used by more than 90% athletes.

3. ***Custom made mouth protectors:*** This is the best choice of a mouth guard because it is prepared by the dentist to offer a perfect fit. It is fabricated on a dental cast.

Care of mouth guard:

- Clean by washing with soap and warm water.
- Before storing, it should be soaked in a mouth rinse.
- It must be kept well ventilated in a plastic box which has holes so that it is kept dry.
- It should be kept away from sunlight.
- No two individual should interchange their mouth guards.

Q.113. According to Freudian psychosexual stages of development the stage which corresponds with development of mixed dentition and character formation is:

1. Concrete operational
2. Latency
3. Phallic
4. Genital

Ans. (2). Latency *(Shobha Tondon 1st ed., P. 123, 124).*

Freud's stage of development:

1. ***Birth (0-1 year):*** It is the first experience to effect personality development.
   - Abrupt change at birth result in psycho-physiological emergency reactions (Protective shell) similar to fear and anxiety.
   - These reactions help the child to learn some adaptive mechanism against anxiety generating stimuli.
   - Neonates who fail to adapt to abrupt changes get started easily. This result in a more protective mechanism which is maladaptive in later life.
2. ***Oral stage (one year):*** In infants the oral cavity is the site for identity needs. It therefore serves as an erogenous zone.
   - This is a dependent stage since the infant is dependent on adults for getting his oral needs fulfilled.
   - If children are not adequately met in this stage the following traits develop.
3. ***Anal stage (1-3 years):*** During this stage maturation of neuromuscular control occurs.

- Control over sphincters particularly anal sphincter result in increased voluntary activity.
- Development of personal autonomy and independence.
- The child realises his control over needs and practices it with a sense of shame or self doubt.
- The child realizes the increasing voluntary control which provides him with the sense of independence and autonomy.
- It is characterized by various abnormal behaviours like disorderliness, abstinence, stubbornness, willfulness, frugality.

Urethral stage: It is a transition between the anal and the phallic stage.

- The child derives pleasure from exercising control over the urinary sphincter.
- The objectives are similar to those of anal stage.
- Loss of urethra control result in shame.

Phallic stage (3-6 years): The stage begins during the 3rd year of life till the 5th year.

- It is characterised by Oedipus complex, castration anxiety, electra complex.
- The child realizes the sexual qualities without embarrassment.
- If the above mentioned characteristics are not resolved the balance between male and female roles does not develop.

Latency stage (6-12 years): Resolution of any defects occur in this phase.

- Maturation of ego takes place.

- The goal of this phase is the further development of personality.
- Lack of inner control of excessive inner control result in a pathological trait.

Genital stage (12-20 years): Psychosexual development extends form 11 to 13 years to young adulthood.

- Sense of identity develops.
- Child has a matured personality.
- Helps to separate from the dependence on parents
- Unresolved traits from previous phases are seen in a modified form.

Q.114. Class II cavity preparation for amalgam restoration in deciduous teeth requires:

1. More buccolingual extension
2. More mesiodistal extension
3. More gingival
4. More cervical

Ans. (1). More buccolingual extensiŏn *(Shobha Tondon 1st ed., P. 288, 289).*

The class II cavity preparation for amalgam restoration in deciduous teeth require more buccolingual extension as the constant point are broad and flat.

Feature of C-II Cavities in deciduous teeth:

- Due to presence of broad contact areas the gingival floor of the proximal box should be wide so as to place the margins in self cleansing areas.
- The box should however converge occlusally with the buccal and lingual wall paralleling the external surface of tooth.
- The wall of proximal box should not be flared as it would lead to unsupported enamel.
- Isthmus width should not exceed 1/3rd the intercuspal width in primary molars.
- Mesiodistally the cusp should not be reduced more than 1/3rd the crown's mesiodistal length.
- Since the enamel rod's at the cervical area of the tooth are oriented occlusally the gingival seat should not be beveled, rather should follow the enamel rod inclination.
- If the depth of the lesion is farther gingivally the axial wall should follow the contour of the

external surface. This will prevent pulp exposure from occurring.

- Proximal box should allow the passage of an explorer tip between its margins and adjacent tooth in all three directions, bucally, gingivally and lingually.

Difficulty encountered in the primary dentition are due to deep cervical constriction, broad contacts and prominent buccal cervical ridges of enamel.

Q.115. The arch length preservation can be best carried out by:

1. Placing a lingual arch
2. Restoring carious teeth
3. Placing band and loop space maintainer
4. Placing an acrylic removable space maintainer.

Ans. (2). Restoring carious teeth *(Rani 3rd ed., P. 192, Bhalajhi 2nd ed., P. 222).*

The deciduous teeth are excellent natural space maintainers until the developing permanent teeth are ready to erupt into the oral cavity.

So caries involving the proximal surface of deciduous teeth if not restored leads to loss of arch length by movement of adjacent teeth into that space. Once caries is detected, proper restoration of the affected teeth should be undertaken immediately to prevent loss of arch length.

(Bhalajhi)

Q.116. In cardiac pulmonary resuscitation chest compressions is done:

1. On the upper part of sternum
2. On the xiphisternum
3. On the middle of the lower part of the sternum
4. On the left side of the chest.

Ans. (3). On the middle of the lower part of the sternum *(Vinod Kapoor 1st ed., P. 485).*

Cardiopulmonary resuscitation: In cardiac arrest, if circulation is absent the external cardiac massage is done for artificial circulation.

- The patient is made to lie on a hard surface preferably on the floor. The rescue sits by the side of the victim.
- The heal of the left hand is placed over the lower half of the sternum just above the xiphisternum and fingers off the chest wall.
- The other hand displaced over it with the arms straight pressure is exerted to depress the sternum by one and a half to two inches by putting on the weight of the rescuer over his hands.
- It compress the heart between the sternum and the spine. The release of pressure allows venous return and refilling of heart.
- The procedure should be carried out at a rate of 60 strokes/min.
- A precardial thump in the form of a sharp single blow with the distance of approximately one foot is known to generate electrical stimulus in the heart. It is recommended as an initial step of resuscitation in monitored patients developing cardiac arrest.

Q.117. The Gillies temporal approach for reduction of zygomatica fracture Rowes zygomatic elevator is placed between:

1. Superficial fascia and temporal fascia
2. Between the temporal bone and the temporatis muscle
3. Between the temporal fascia and the temporalis muscle
4. Skin and superficial fascia

Ans. (3). Between the temporal fascia and the temporalis muscle *(Vinod Kapoor 1st ed., P. 258).*

In Gillie's approach 2 cm long incision is made parallel to the anterior branch of superficial temporal artery. This is normally at an angle of 45 degree to the zygomatic arch. Dissection is carried out to expose the glistening white temporal fascia. Then the fascia is incised and the temporalis muscle comes into view. Zygomatic bone elevator is pushed between the temporal fascia and temporalis muscle to engage the zygmatic bone or arch. The zygomatic bone or arch can be lifted. Iodoform roll gauze can be packed behind the zygomatic bone for 5-7 days. Then suturing is done.

Q.118. In which one of the following conditions the sialography is contraindicated?

1. Ductal calculus
2. Chronic parotitis
3. Acute parotitis
4. Recurrent sialadenitis

Ans. (3). Acute parotitis *(Vinod Kapoor 1st ed., P. 308, 309).*

Sialography: is a radiographic feature that is useful diagnostic adjunct for the detection and monitoring of salivary gland disease. In this technique some dye is injected in the salivary gland and the radiographs of these glands are taken to study normal anatomy, physiology or any pathologic condition in relation to the gland. These radiographs are called sialograph or sialograms.

Indication:

1. To study normal anatomy and physiologic function of the gland or any shrinkage or obstruction of the duct etc.
2. To study any pathologic conditions like inflammation, stones, sialoliths, space occupying lesion (benign tumour or malignancies), strictures of the duct.

Agent used: Iodinated contrast media (dyes are lipid soluble - Lipoidal or water soluble - Hyopaque).

Administration: Retrograde pressure placement of contrast media into the major duct.

Amount: 0.75-1 ml for submandibular gland
1-1.5 ml for parotid gland.

Detector: Fluoroscope and X-ray film.

Structure visualised: Ductal system, one major salivary gland visualised at a time.

Advantage:

1. High resolution of the ductal system.
2. Controlled localised radiation dose.
3. Much information on appearance of specific disease state.

Contraindications:

1. When patient is allergic to iodine.
2. In case of fulminating ascending infection of the gland from the ductal opening.

Radiographs: Lateral oblique or PA views.

Interpretation of the finding:

1. ***Normal gland:*** appears as a leafless tree.
2. ***Inflammation/blockage:*** Some buds are seen on the branches/offshoot e.g. in sialadenitis.
3. ***Strictures:*** Post contraction dialation (a sausage defect seen).
4. ***Growth:*** If tumour is benign
   - Localised filling defect
   - If malignant - spillage defect (Scattered dye)
5. ***Stone:*** A filling defect distal to the obstruction.

Q.119. A woman with infertility receives an ovary transplant from her sister who is an identical twin. What type of graft it is:

1. Xenograft
2. Autograft
3. Allograft
4. Isograft

Ans. (4). Isograft *(Ananthnarayan 6th ed., P. 164).*

Types of Grafts:

1. ***Autograft:*** Graft taken from some individual from one anatomical site to the other.
2. ***Homograft or allograft:*** Graft taken from an individual of the same species who is not genetically related.
3. ***Isograft (synergic graft):*** When the graft has been derived from an individual having the same genetic disposition e.g. identical twins.
4. ***Heterograft or Xenograft:*** When graft has been derived from donor of another species.
5. ***Alloplast:*** These are graft which are nonbiological materials like metallic alloys, synthetic polymers and rubber etc.
6. ***Orthotropic graft:*** A transplant placed in its normal anatomic site.
7. ***Heterotopic graft:*** A transplant placed in a site, different to that where the organ is normally located.

Q.120. The drug of choice in management of a patient with an acute allergic reaction involving bronchospasm and hypotension is:

1. Epinephrine
2. Aminophyline
3. Dexamethasone
4. Diphenhydramine

Ans. (1). Epinephrine *(Vinod Kapoor 1st ed., P. 481-483).*

Epinephrine is used because it cause bronchodialation and relieves from hypotension.

When bronchospasm occur there is generalised contractions of smooth muscle of the bronchial tree. In an asthmatic attack, bronchospasm leads to airflow obstruction which is aggravated by oedema of the lining as well as collection of secretions in bronchioles giving a radiological picture of consolidation. There is dyspnoea or orthopnoea, wheezing is a prominent sign which means forced respiration due to bronchial narrowing. Wheezing is localised in bronchial obstruction. There is shortness of breathing, wheezing and tightness in the chest. As the attacks prolongs symptoms of fatigue, restlessness and irritability appear. It may be accompanied by cyanosis with the accessory muscle showing laboured breathing along with suprasternal and intercostal retraction.

Management:

1. Patient is allowed to sit down in a reclining posture.
2. 100% oxygen is administered if cyanosis has

established otherwise 20-30% oxygen is extremely useful.

3. Injection aminophylline 5-6 mg/kg body weight should be given intravenously.
4. Steroids like hydrocortisone hemi-succinate or dexamethasone may be given intravenously as life saving drug.
5. Injection of adrenaline 0.3 mg (1:1000 dilution is given subcutaneously in status asthmatics.
6. Mucolytic agent like bromohexine along with steam inhalation and cover of antibiotics are important in the management.

In case of hypotension:

1. Put the patient in supine position with legs raised. Patient with cardiac ailment should be placed in semi-sitting position.
2. 100% O_2 should be administered.
3. IV line should immediately be maintained with ringer lactate solution.
4. Atropine 0.6 mg diluted in 5 ml of sterile water is given intravenously slowly if the pulse is less than 60 per min.
5. Injection mephenterimine 15 mg can be administered intravenously or intramuscularly. At times phenylephrine 2 mg subcutaneously is also recom-mended.
6. Hydrocortisone sodium succinate 100 mg should be administered intra-venously for combating stress.

Q.121. The agent of choice to reverse status epilepticus by local anaesthetic overdose is:

1. Oxygen
2. Diazepam
3. Epinephrine
4. Phenobarbital

Ans. (2). Diazepam *(Malamed, Emergencies in Dental Office 1st ed., P. 326, 327).*

- Local anaesthetic overdose cause status epilepticus. So anti-convulsant drug is used. Oral route is contraindicated in unconscious, convulsing patients. The drug should be injected directly into veins. Because the blood pressure is elevated significantly during the seizure, superficial peripheral veins usually are visible, which makes injection relatively easy for an experienced doctor who has an assistant to restrain the arm.
- The anti-convulsant drug mostly used is benzodiazepine, either diazepam (valium) or midazolam. Diazepam is 90% effective in instance of primary convulsive status.
- A 10 mg dose should be administered at a rate of 5 mg per minute and repeated every 10 minute, as necessary.
- Children receive diazepam in dose of 0.3 mg/kg, a dose that should be repeated every 10 minute, as necessary. The total dose should not exceed 0.5 mg/kg for acute therapy.

Management of generalised convulsive status epilepticus

(Prodromal stage)

Terminate dental procedure

↓

(Ictal stage)

Position patient supine with the legs elevated slightly

↓

Summon emergency medical assistance

Airway, breathing, circulation - Asses and perform basic life support

↓

Definite care

Protect patient from injury

Administer O_2

Monitor vital signs

↓

If seizure persists for more than 5 minutes

↓

Airway, breathing, circulation basic life support

↓

Protect patient until medical assistance arrive

↓

Perform venipuncture and administer Perform anticonvulsant drug via IV route

↓

Administer a 50% dextrose solution via IV route provide subsequent management (hospitalization)

Q.122. Mucoperiosteal flaps:

1. When raised do not cause postoperative swelling and pain
2. Are raised whenever bone removal is desired to facilitate extraction.
3. Are routinely raised during extraction
4. When raised will cause trauma and injury to underlying osseus tissues.

Ans. (2). Are raised whenever bone removal is desired to facilitate extraction *(Vinod Kapoor 1st ed., P. 39)*.

- Mucoperiosteal flap is raised during surgical extraction of tooth. The reflection of adequate mucoperiosteal flap is done and removal of bone followed by removal of tooth is done. In multirooted tooth the division of tooth is indicated.
- The advantage of open extraction involve removal of teeth lying in difficult positions without damaging the neurovascular bundle. The fracture of bone are avoided. There is less danger of creating an oroantral fistula and there are less chance of tearing of soft tissue and fracture of large piece of alveolar bone.

The mucoperiosteal flap is raised when

1. Any tooth resist extraction by closed method.
2. Unerupted tooth which can not be removed by closed method.
3. Fractured tooth or roots below the level of epithelial attachment.
4. Teeth with hypercementosis of roots.
5. Teeth with fused, dilacerated and locked roots.

6. Teeth with widely divergent roots.
7. Teeth with complicated and unfavourbale root curvature.
8. Teeth with post crowns or very large root canal fillings.
9. Roots which are dipping into the maxillary antrum.
10. Ankylosed roots especially in elderly persons.
11. When there is a danger of fracture of the alveolar or basal bone.

Q.123. The proper rate of rescue breathing in an adult is:

1. 4 times per minute
2. 12 times per minute
3. 20 times per minute
4. 28 times per minute

Ans. (2).12 times per minute *(Vinod Kapoor 1st ed., P. 485, Malamed emergency in dental office 1st ed., P. 486, 487).*

- In the absence of effective respiratory movement artificial ventilation must be started immediately.
- To perform mouth to mouth ventilation, head tilt must be maintained and the nose of the victim sealed.
- The first ventilatory cycle is composed of two full ventilation with adequate time (1½ to 2 seconds per breath) allowed to provide good chest expansion and to minimize the risk of gastric distention.
- Effective artificial ventilation is noted by expansion of the victim's chest. In normal adult, the minimal volume of air should be 800 ml/breath but need not exceed 1200 ml/breath for adequate ventilation.
- Subsequent ventilation are performed at a rate of one every 5 seconds (12 times per minute) for adult victim.
- In the child and infant, ventilation is carried out at a rate of one every 3 seconds (20 per minute), with each breath lasting approximately 1 to 1½ seconds.
- Immediately after the first ventilatory cycle of two full breaths, the rescuer determine the victims cardiovascular status.

Q.124. A dermatome is used:

1. To remove scar tissue
2. To harvest skin graft
3. To abrade skin which is pigmented
4. For pairing of lacerated soft tissue

Ans. (2). To harvest skin graft *(Vinod Kapoor 1st ed., P. 408).*

- Full thickness or split thickness grafts are used from forearm or thigh region. Split skin grafts are harvested with the help of dermatome to be transplanted intraorally especially in the management of oral submucous fibrosis or carcinoma in situ. Full thickness grafts alongwith part of pecroalis muscle or deltoid muscle is used as a pedicle graft for restoration of contour and cosmetics of maxillofacial region especially in oncology. Also used for reconstruction purposes are the forehead or scalp flap and tubed pedicle flaps from the thoracoepigastric region.
- Free dermal graft with or without underlying fat are harvested from forearm or thigh. A dermatose is used for the purpose.

Q.125. The rate of injection of intravenous volium is:

1. 1 ml/min
2. 2.5 ml/min
3. 1 mg/min
4. 2.5 mg/min

Ans. (1).1 ml/min *(Vinod Kapoor 1st ed., P. 400).*

Valium: It is the most commonly used sedative, can be given through oral, intravascular or intravenous route. It is fairly safe drug. Normally 10 mg dose is sufficient for healthy adult individual. For intravenous route 2 ml ampule with 5 mg/ml diazepam is available. The injection should be given slowly at the rate of 1 ml/min and should be administered in a large vein. It can be given along with intravenous infusion of Ringer Lactate solution. A maximum dose of 20 mg should not be exceeded. The patient is not allowed to walk around postoperatively without attendant. Automobile driving is strictly not allowed. Diazepam can be combined with Pentazocine Lactate (Fortwin) to potentiate the sedation and analgesia.

Q.126. The longest acting local anaesthetic is:

1. Prilocaine
2. Lignocaine
3. Bupivacaine
4. Ropivacaine

Ans. (3). Bupivacaine *(Malamed Book of Local Anaesthesia 4th ed., P. 288 Monheim LA 7th ed., P. 157).*

Long acting LA (180 min. or longer)	**Short acting LA** (45-75 min.)	**Ultra short acting LA** (less than 30 min.)
Dibucaine	2% Lidocaine with vasoconstrictor	Lidocaine (plain)
Bupivacaine	4% prilocaine with vasoconstrictor	Prilocaine
Etidocaine	2% Procaine with vasoconstrictor	Procaine 2 Chlorprocaine

Indications of Bupivacaine:

1. Lengthy dental procedure for which pulpal (deep) anaesthesia in excess of 90 min is required e.g. full mouth reconstruction, implant surgery and extensive periodontal.
2. Management of postoperative pain (e.g. endodontic periodontal and surgical).

C/I: Bupivacaine is not recommended in younger patients or in those for whom the risk of postoperative soft tissue injury produced by self-mutilation is increased such as physically and mentally in children because paediatric dental procedure are usually of short duration.

Read text below:

Ropivacaine: is a long acting amide anesthetic,

similar to bupivacaine and etidocaine in duration of activity. It is similar structurally to mepivacaine and bupivacaine but is unique in that ropivacaine is prepared as an isomer rather than as a racemic mixture, have lower arrhythmogenic potential than bupivacaine. The half life of ropivacaine is 25.9 min which is shorter than that of other amides. Ropivacaine has decreased cardiotoxicity relative to bupivacaine but its clinical duration of action is approximately 20% shorter. The primary use of ropivacaine in anaesthesiology has been for regional nerve block, primarily epidural. Its potential for use in dentistry as another long acting local anaesthetic appears great but awaits clinical evaluation.

Mol. wt. - 274

Pka - 8.1

Q.127. Amide-type local anaesthetics are metabolised in the:

1. Serum
2. Liver
3. Spleen
4. Kidneys

Ans. (2). Liver *(Malamed, Local anaesthesia 4th ed., P. 27, 28)*

Metabolism of amide:

- The metabolism of the amide local anaesthetics is more complex than that of esters.
- Primary site of bio-transformation of amide drug is the liver.
- Virtually the entire metabolic process occur in the liver for lidocaine, mepivacaine, articaine, etidocaine, bupivacaine.
- Prilocaine undergoes primary metabolism in the liver with some also possibly occurring in lung.
- Prilocaine undergoes more rapid biotransformation than the other amides.
- 70% of a dose of infected lidocaine undergo biotransformation in patients with normal liver function. Patient with lower than usual hepatic blood flow (hypotensive, congestive heart failure) or poor liver function (cirrhosis) are unable to biotransform amide local anaesthetic at a normal rate. This slower than normal biotransformation rate leads to increased anaesthetic blood levels and potentially increase toxicity.
- Patient receiving large dose prilocaine or articaine can develop methaemoglobinemia.
- Prilocaine the parent compound, can not produce methaemoglobinemia but orthotoluidine,

a primary metabolite of prilocaine does induce the formation of methaemoglobin, which is responsible for methaemoglobinemia if methaemoglobin blood levels become elevated.

Q.128. Nitrous oxide is a colourless, sweet smelling gas with a density of:

1. 1.5
2. 0.5
3. 2.5
4. 3.5

Ans. (1).1.5 *(Ajay Yadav 1st ed., P. 57).*

Nitrous oxide: Also called as laughing gas:

- Name given by Humphry Davy
- It was first prepared by Joseph Pristley in 1774.

Preparation: Prepared by heating ammonium nitrate between 245-270°C.

Physical properties: It is colourless, non irritating and sweet smelling.

- Boiling point is –89°C.
- Critical temperature is 36.5°C which is above room temperature therefore it can be kept in liquified state.
- Stored as liquid in blue colour cylinder (Cylinder pressure 760 Psi)
- Mol. wt. 44.
- 1.5 times heavier than air (density 1.527).
- 35 times more soluble than nitrogen.
- Blood gas coefficient is 0.47
- Usually given in mixture of nitrous oxide 66% and oxygen 33%)
- Impurities present in cylinder can cause severe laryngospasm, methaemoglobinemia, pulmonary oedema.

Systemic action: CVS - depress myocardium

- Cerebral - Raise intracranial tension

- Respiratory system - Cause tachypnea, decrease tidal volume
- Immunologic system - Effect chemotaxis and motility of leukocytes.

Side Effect: Haematological system - cause bone marrow depression, cause aplastic and megaloblastic anaemia.

Neurological system: subacute degeneration of spinal cord.

Germ cell: increased risk of abortion.

Contraindication: C/I in

1. Pneumothorax
2. Pneumoperitoneum
3. Pneumocephalum
4. Middle ear surgery and tympanoplasties
5. Posterior fossa surgeries
6. Laproscopic surgeries
7. Acute intestinal obstruction and volvulus of gut
8. Eye surgeries

Use in anaesthesia:

1. As a supplement to anaesthesia.
2. As a carrier gas for inhalation agents.
3. As analgesics in obstetrics, dental pain, burn dressing, acute trauma.

Q.129. The first drug of choice to be administered for anaphylaxis is:

1. Hydrocortisone
2. Adrenaline
3. Atropine
4. Chlorpheneramine maleate

Ans. (2). Adrenaline *(K.D. Tripathi 5th ed., P. 63).*

Anaphylactic reactions: Reaginic antibodies (IgE) are produced which get fixed to the mast cell. On exposure to drug, antigen antibody reaction takes place on the mast cell surface releasing mediators like histamine, 5-HT, leukotrienes, specially LTC4, LTD4, prostaglandins, PAF etc. resulting in urticaria, itching, angioedema, asthma, rhinitis, anaphylactic shock. The manifestation occur quickly after challenge and are called immediate hypersensitivity.

Treatment: Inject adrenaline 0.5 mg (0.5 ml of 1 in 1000 solution) im, repeat every 5-10 min in case patient does not improve or improvement is transient. This is only life saving measure.

Adrenaline should not be injected i.v. (can itself be fatal) unless shock is immediately life threatening. It adrenaline is to be injected i.v., it should be diluted to 1:10000 or 1:100000 and infused slowly with constant monitoring.

Q.130. The most common site of leak in CSF rhinorrhoea is

1. Sphenoid sinus
2. Frontal sinus
3. Cribriform plate
4. Tegmen tympani

Ans. (3). Cribriform plate *(Vinod Kapoor 1st ed., P. 239, Logan Turner 10th ed., P. 28, Dhingra 2nd ed., P. 165).*

Fracture of cribriform plate of ethmoid and involvement of ant. cranial fossa result in CSF leak. It poses a serious danger of infection. CSF leak through a dural tear of less than 5 mm diameter stops on reducing the fracture.

Difference between CSF rhinorrhoea and allergic or vasomotor rhinitis.

1. CSF contains glucose which can be demonstrated by chemical tests.
2. CSF when collected into a test tube and allowed to stand, it remains clear in contradistinction to nasal discharge that leaves a sediment because of mucus and other proteins.
3. Nasal discharge stiffens the hand-kerchief and CSF dries soft in it.

Treatment of CSF rhinorrhoea

- **Early post traumatic cases**
- **Early cases of post traumatic CSF rhinorrhoea are treated conservatively**
  - **Patient is placed in semi prone position.**
  - **Avoid blowing of nose, sneezing, straining**
  - **Prophylactic antibiotics administered to prevent meningitis**

- **Persistent case**
- **Persistent case of CSF rhinorrhoea are treated surgically by extracranial or intra-cranial approach**

Q.131. Gracey Curette No. 11-12 are used for:

1. Anterior teeth
2. Posterior teeth mesial
3. Posterior teeth distal
4. Posterior teeth facial and lingual.

Ans. (2). Posterior teeth mesial *(Carranza 9th ed., P. 573).*

- Double-ended Gracey Curettes are paired in the following manner
- Gracey # 1-2 and 3-4 - Anterior teeth.
- Gracey # 5-6 - Anterior teeth and premolars.
- Gracey # 7-8 and 9-10 - Posterior teeth : facial and lingual
- Gracey # 11-12 - Posterior teeth : mesial
- Gracey # 13-14 - Posterior teeth :distal.

Recent addition to the Gracey Curette set have been the Gracey # 15-16 and 17-18. The Gracey # 15-16 is a modification of the standard 11-12 and is designed for mesial surface of posterior teeth. It consist of a Gracey # 11-12 blade combined with the more acutely angled # 13-14 shank. The new shank angulation of the Gracey # 15-16 allows better adaptation to posterior mesial surface from a front position with intraoral rests.

The Gracey # 17-18 is a modification of the # 13-14. It has a terminal shank elongated by 3 mm and a more accentuated angulation of the shank to provide complete occlusal clearance.

Q.132. A black line on the gingival which follows the contour of the margin is due to:

1. Lead
2. Argyria
3. Iron
4. Mercury

Ans. (4). Mercury *(Carranza 9th ed., P. 273).*

- Heavy metals Gismuth, arsenic, mercury lead silver absorbed systematically from therapeutic use of occupational or household environments may discolour the gingival and other areas of the oral mucosal.
- They produce a black line in the gingiva that follows the contour of margin.
- The pigmentation may also appear as isolated black blotches involving the interdental, marginal and attached gingiva. This is different from tattooing produced by accidental embedding of malgam or other metal fragments.
- Gingival pigmentation from systematically absorbed metals result from perivascualr precipitation of metallic sulfide in the sub-epithelial connective tissue.
- It occur only in area of inflammation where the increased permeability of irritated blood vessel permit seepage of metal in to surrounding tissue.

Q.133. Conditional gingival enlargement is usually not:

1. Hormonal
2. Leukemic
3. Granuloma pyogenicum
4. Drug induced

Ans. (4). Drug induced *(Carranza 9th ed., P. 279).*

Gingival enlargement can be classified as:

a. **Inflammatory enlargement:**
   - Chronic
   - Acute

b. **Drug induced enlargement:**

c. **Enlargement associated with systemic disease:**
   - Conditioned enlargement
   - Pregnancy
   - Puberty
   - Vitamin C deficiency
   - Plasma cell gingivitis
   - Non-specific conditioned enlargement (granuloma pyogenicum)
   - Systemic disease causing gingival enlargement
   - Leukemia
   - Granulomatous disease (Wegner's granulomatosis, sarcoidosis)

d. **Neoplastic enlargement (Gingival tumor):**
   - Benign tumors
   - Malignant tumors

e. **False enlargement:**

Q.134. The serum concentration of which of the following human IgG subclass is maximum:

1. IgG_1
2. IgG_2
3. IgG_3
4. IgG_4

Ans. (1).IgG_1 (*Carranza 9th ed., P. 129, Ananthnarayan 6th ed., P. 83*).

Selected Properties of Immunoglobulin Isotypes

Immunoglobulin Isotype	IgG_1	IgG_2	IgG_3	IgG_4	IgM	IgA_1	IgA_2	IgD	IgE
Concentration in serum (mg/ml)	9	3	1	0.5	1.5	3	0.5	0.03	0.00005
Molecular weight (kilodaltons)	146	146	170	146	970	160	160	184	188

Q.135. Glucose levels in gingival crevicular fluid (GCF) are:

1. Equal to glucose level in serum
2. Zero
3. 3-4 times greater than serum levels
4. More than 10 times the serum levels

Ans. (3).3-4 times greater than serum levels *(Carranza 9th ed., P. 257).*

Gingival Crevicular Fluid:

Organic compounds: Both carbohydrates and protein are found in GCF. Glucose hexosamine and hexuronic acid are two of the compounds in GCF.

- Glucose concentration in GCF is 3-4 times greater than that in serum
- The total protein content of GCF is much less than that of serum.
- Metabolic and bacterial products identified in GCF include lactic acid, urea, hydroproline, endotoxins, cytotoxic substances hydrogen sulfide and antibacterial factors.

Method for analysis of GCF:

- Fluorometry for the detection of metalloprotease
- ELISA test to detect enzyme levels and IL-1B.
- Radioimmunoassays to detect cyclooxygenase derivatives and procollagen III.
- Timidazole detected by high pressure liquid chromatography.
- Acute phase proteins detected by direct and indirect immunodots and others.

GCF production is increased by mastication of coarse foods, tooth brushing and gingival massage, ovulation, hormonal contraceptives and smoking, circardian periodicity and periodontal therapy.

Q.136. The oxygen consumption of normal gingiva is:

1. 1.6 ± 0.37
2. 0.9 ± 0.22
3. 2.7 ± 0.41
4. 1.9 ± 0.21

Ans. (1).1.6 ± 0.37 Ref. Still searching.

This question is given in some MCQ books and the answer is (1) is confirmed.

Q.137. Salivary pellicle is composed of the following except:

1. Immunoglobulin G
2. Immunoglobulin A
3. Amylase
4. Albumin

Ans. (4). Albumin *(Carranza 9th ed., P. 259).*

- Immunoglobulin IgG and IgM are present but the predominant immunoglobulin found in saliva is IgA. IgG is more prevalent in GCF.
- Major and minor salivary gland contribute all the secretory IgA and lesser amount of IgG and IgM.
- IgA antibodies present in parotid saliva can inhibit the attachment of oral streptococcus species to epithelial cells.
- Antibodies in the secretions may impair the ability of bacteria to attack to mucosal or ductal surface.
- The enzyme fond in saliva are derived from the salivary gland, bacteria leukocytes, oral tissues and ingested substances.
- The major enzyme is parotid amylase.
- Glycoproteins selectively adsorb to the hydroxyapatite to make up part of the acquired pellicle.
- Other salivary glycoproteins inhibit the sorption of some bacteria to the tooth surface and to epithelial cells of the oral mucosal.

Q.138. The characteristic lesion of acute necrotizing gingivitis is the necrosis of the gingival mainly of the:

1. Interdental papilla
2. Marginal gingiva
3. Attached gingiva
4. Free gingiva

Ans. (1). Interdental papilla *(Carranza 9th ed., P. 298)*.

Pindborg have described the following stages in the progress of NUG.

1. Only the tip of the interdental papilla is affected.
2. The lesion extends to marginal gingiva and cause punched out papilla.
3. The attached gingiva is also affected.
4. Bone is exposed.

Horning and Cohen extended the staging of these oral necrotizing disease as follows:

Stage I – Necrosis of the tip of the interdental papilla (93%).

Stage II – Necrosis of the entire papilla (19%)

Stage III – Necrosis extending to the gingival margin (21%).

Stage IV – Necrosis extending also to the attached gingiva (1%).

Stage V – Necrosis extending into buccal or labial mucosa (6%).

Stage VI – Necrosis exposing alveolar bone (1%).

Stage VII – Necrosis perforating skin of cheek (0%).

Q.139. The normal depth of the gingival crevica in an adult does not exceed:

1. 0.5-1 mm
2. 1-2 mm
3. 1-3 mm
4. 2-3 mm

Ans. (4).2-3 mm *(Carranza 9th ed., P. 17).*

The gingival crevice is the shallow crevice or space around the tooth bounded by the surface of the tooth on one side and the epithelial lining the free gingiva of the gingiva on the other. It is V shape. The depth of this sulcus as determined in histologic section has been reported as 1.8 mm with variation from 0-6 mm. The depth of gingival sulcus is measured by periodontal probe. The histologic depth of a sulcus need not be exactly equal to the depth of peneration of the probe. The so called probing depth of a clinically normal gingival sulcus in humans is 2-3 mm.

Q.140. Embrasure characterized by a slight to moderate session of interdental papilla are:

1. Type I
2. Type II
3. Type III
4. Type IV

Ans. (2). Type II *(Carranza 8th ed., P. 502, Satish Chandra 1st ed., P. 117).*

Type I – No gingival recession - use dental floss.

Type II – Moderate papillary recession - use interdental brush

Type III – Complete loss of papillae - Use unitufted brush.

(Carranza 8th ed.)

Type of embrasure	Condition of gingiva in the embrasure	Cleaning aid recommended for the embrasure cleansing
I	Embrasure are completely occupied by healthy interdental papilla.	Superfine and thin dental floss used only for cleaning sulcus.
II	About 75% of embrasure is occupied by gingiva	Medium or coarse and thick dental floss
III	About 50% of the embrasure is occupied by the gingiva	Thin fine pointed small spiral interdental brushes
IV	About 25% of the embrasure is occupied by the gingiva	Thick spiral interdental brushes and fine or thin bristles ended unitufted brushes.
V	Complete loss of interdental papilla and gingiva from the embrasure the level of the gingiva in the interdental space is same as the buccal and lingual gingiva on the teeth.	Bristles ended unitufted brushes and thick spiral interdental brushes

(Satish Chandra 1st ed.)

Q.141. Most recent type of deuture adhesive is:

1. Salt of Gontrez
2. Natural gums
3. Cellulose based salt
4. Acrylic adhesives

Ans. (1). Salt of gontrez *(Boucher 12th ed., P. 443)*.

- Denture adhesive materials in use before the early 1960s were based on vegetable gums (e.g. Karaya, tragacanth, xanthan and acacia) that play modest, nonionic adhesion to both denture and mucosal and possessed very little cohesive strength. Gum based adhesives (still commercially available are highly water soluble, particularly in hot liquids such a coffee, tea, and soups and therefore washed out readily from beneath dentures.
- The most popular and successful products consist of mixtures of the salt of short acting (CMC) and long acting (polyvinylmethyl ethermaleate) or "Gantrez" polymers. In the presence of water CMC hydrates and displays quick onset ionic adherence to both dentures and mucous epithelium. The original fluid increase its viscocity and CMC increase in volume thereby eliminating voids between prosthesis and basal seat.
- Gantrez salt hydrate and increase adherence and viscocity. The long acting (i.e. less soluble) Gantrez salt also display molecular cross linking resulting in measurable increase incohesive behaviour.

Q.142. Face bow is used to transfer:

1. Axis orbital plane
2. Frankfort horizontal plane
3. Camper plane
4. Occlusal plane

Ans. (1). Axis orbital plane *(Boucher 11th ed., P. 198)*.

Face bow: The face bow is a caliper like device that is used to record the relationship of the jaws to the temporomandibular joints or the opening axis of the jaws and to orient the cast in this same relationship to the opening axis of the articulator.

Arbitrary face bow is placed on the face with the condyle rods located approximately over the condyle.

Kinematic face bow is so designed that the opening axis of the mandible can be located more accurately.

In arbitrary face bow the condyle rods of one particular model are positioned on a line extending from the outer canthus to the top of the tragus and approximately 13 mm in front of the external auditory meatus. This placement generally locate the rods within 5 mm of the true center of the opening axis of the jaws. Face bow are used to orient cast on an articulator in the same relation to the opening axis of the articulator as the jaws are the opening axis of the mandible.

The use of face bow is predicted on an arbitrary location of the opening axis of the mandible.

Q.143. Beyron point is located at:

1. 13 mm anterior to posterior margin of tragus on a line from center of tragus to outer canthus.
2. 11 mm anterior to posterior margin of tragus on a line from parallel to and 7 mm below FHP.
3. 10 mm anterior to posterior margin of tragus on a line from center of tragus to outer canthus.
4. 13 mm anterior to tragus on a line from base of tragus to outer canthus.

Ans. (1).13 mm anterior to posterior margin of tragus on a line from center of tragus to outer canthus *(Nallaswamy 1st ed., P. 125, 127)*.

Arbitrary Methods

Arbitrary Hinge axis points	Accuracy percentage	Investigator
13 mm anterior to posterior margin of tragus to the outer canthus	98.0 92.1 58.3	Schall horn Beyron Beck
13 mm in front of anterior margin of meatus	16.7 40.0	Beck Lauritzen & Lundeen
13 mm from foot of tragus to canthus	33.0	Teteruck and Lundeen
10 mm anterior to center of external auditory meatus and 7 mm below Frankfort plane	83.3	Beck
Ear axis	75.5	Teteruck and Lundeen

Note: A 5 mm deviation from the hinge axis can result in a minute error of 0.2 mm at the 2nd molar (Weinberg). This error is insignificant for most CD, RPD, FPD procedure.

Q.144. Denture stability refers to resistance of a denture:

1. To move in a vertical direction away from basal seat
2. To move in a vertical direction forward basal seat
3. To movements its tissue foundation especially to lateral force.
4. Against any kind of movement more than 25 μm in any direction.

Ans. (3). To movements its tissue foundation especially to lateral force *(Boucher 10th ed., P. 169, 171 Nallaswamy 1st ed., P. 64).*

Stability of a denture its quality of being steady and constant in position when force are applied to it stability refers especially to resistance against horizontal movement and force that tend to alter the relationship between the denturebase and its supporting foundation in a horizontal or rotatory direction. Stability depend on following factor.

- Size and form of the basal seat.
- The quality of final impressions.
- The form of the polished surfaces
- The proper location
- Arrangement of the artificial teeth.

Retention for a denture is its resistance to removal in a direction opposite that of its insertion. It is the quality inherent in a denture that resist the force of the gravity, the adhesiveness of foods, the forces associated with the opening the jaws. Retention is the means by which denture are held in position in the mouth.

Support is the resistance of adenture to the vertical components of mastication and to occlusal or other forces applied in a direction forward to the basal seat. Support is provided by the maxillary and mandibular bones and their covering of mucosal tissues. It is enhanced by selective placement of pressures that are in hormony with the resiliency of the tissue that make up the basal seat.

Q.145. During Bennett movement or shift of mandible:

1. Condyle of working side exhibit bodily forward movement.
2. Condyle of non-working side exhibit bodily lateral movement.
3. Condyle of working side exhibit bodily lateral movement.
4. Condyle of working side exhibit bodily lateral and forward movement.

Ans. (3).Condyle of working side exhibit bodily lateral movement *(Vimal Sikri 1st ed., P. 39, Boucher 11th ed., P. 221,276).*

Bennett shift is the lateral bodily shift of mandible towards the working side in function and occurs to some extent in most patients during lateral functional movements. The amount and the timing of lateral shift influence the pattern of tooth contact during lateral excursion. The direction and travel of mandibular posterior cusps in influenced by amount and timing of Bennett shift.

(Vimal Sikri)

- According to the finding of Gysi, 15 degree is the average Bennett Shift (Dr. Normann Bennett, 1908)
- The magnitude of the shift in normal TMJ varies from 0-1.5 mm.

Bennett angle: the angle formed by the Saggital plane and the path of advancing Condyle during lateral mandibular movements.

Bennett angle (L) = (H/8) + 12

H is height of Condylar inclination.

Average Bennettangle 15 degree.

More about Bennett shift: Bennett shift can be of following types.

Progressive side shift: The orbiting Condyle may follow a pathway which plots a straight line, when the shift is distributed throughout the range of motion called as progressive side shift.

Precurrent shift: It may follow a pathway when the lateral shift occur in first 2 or 3 mm of forward movement and is called precurrent shift.

Immediate side shift: When shift occur before any forward movement of the orbiting Condyle. So the pathway will be almost straight; mesially in some direction as to shift of rotating Condyle without any component of forward movement.

Q.146. To increase resistance form of an excessively tapered preparation:

1. Reduce height of preparation to shorten arc of rotation
2. Increase cervical reduction to taper
3. Add groove
4. Use adhesive cement.

Ans. (3). Add groove *(Rosenstiel 3rd ed., P. 188, 189)*.

- The tooth preparation must be so shaped that particular areas of axial wall will prevent rotation of the crown.
- Increase preparation taper and rounding of axial angles tend to reduce resistance. Short tooth preparations with large diameters were found to have very little resistance form.
- Resistance is greater if these have walls that are perpendicular to the direction of the applied force.
- Thus U shaped grooves or flared boxes provided more resistance than do V shaped one.
- Resistance form of an excessively taper preparation can be improved by adding mesiodistal groove or pinholes, because these interfere with rotational movement.
- In a short or excessively tapered complete crown resistance form is minimal because most of the buccal wall is missing. A mesiodistal groove should be placed to increase resistance form.

Q.147. The posterior tooth that gives a better support is:

1. With convergent roots
2. Divergent roots
3. Conical roots
4. Curved roots

Ans. (2).Divergent roots *(Rosenstiel 3rd ed., P. 71).*

- When tooth support is borderline, the shape of the roots and their angulation should be considered.
- A molar with divergent roots will provide better support than a molar with conical roots and little or no interradicular bone.
- A single rooted tooth with an elliptic cross section will offer better support than a tooth with similar root surface area but a circular cross section.
- A well aligned tooth will provide better support than a tilted one.

Q.148. A pier abutment is:

1. Periodontal weak abutment
2. With an edentulous space on both side of the abutment
3. Edentulous space on one side of the abutment
4. Abutment adjacent to edentulous space.

Ans. (2). With an edentulous space on both side of the abutment *(Nallaswamy 1st ed., P. 525)*.

Pier abutment:

- At pier abutment is one with edentulous spaces present on either side. In such cases a single prosthesis is fabricated using all three abutments.
- The central (pier) abutment is subjected to leverage and tortional forces acting on the different parts of denture.
- In order to protect the pier abutment, specially designed fixed partial dentures using non-rigid connectors have been proposed.

Q.149. Minimal occlusal clearance on centric cusp for cast metal is:

1. 0.5 mm
2. 1 mm
3. 1.5 mm
4. 2 mm

Ans. (3).1.5 mm *(Rosenstiel 3rd ed., P. 21, 204, 205).*

Following are the criteria for cast metal crown:

1. Minimum clearance on non-centric cusp is 1 mm.
2. Minimum clearance on centric cusp is 1.5 mm.
3. Chamfer width 0.5 mm.
4. Taper 6 degree.

Functional (centric) cusp bevel: Proper tooth preparation for a complete cast crown will result in the reduction being directly beneath the cusp of crown. This is important for ensuing optimum restoration contour with maximum durability and conservation of tooth structure. Proper placement of functional cusp bevel will achieve it. Because additional reduction is needed for functional cusp (to give 1.5 mm occlusal clearance), the bevel must be angled flatter than the external surface. On most teeth the functional cusp bevel will be placed at about 45 degree to long axis.

Q.150. Important diagnostic tool for achieving accurate implant angulation:

1. Diagnostic template
2. Wax up
3. Mounted diagnostic cast
4. Surgical template

Ans. (4).Surgical template *(Rosensteil 3rd ed., P. 323, 325).*

- Surgical guide template is extremely useful for anterior implants because slight variations in angulation can significantly affect the appearance of the final restoration.
- Construction of surgical guide template has become a requirement in those patients in whom it is necessary to optimize fixed replacements and ensure correct emergence profiles.
- Surgical templates can also be beneficial in areas where esthetics is less important.

The objective for using a surgical template in partially edentulour patients are as follows.

1. Delineate the embrasures
2. Locate the implant within the restoration contour.
3. Align implants within the long axis of the completed restoration.
4. Identify the level of the CEJ or tooth emergence from the soft tissue.
   - This type of template is fabricated from a diagnostic waxing and denture tooth arrangement on a mounted cast.
   - The use of surgical guide template is most necessary in maxillary anterior region, were bony dimensions are sometime surprising

and often unfavourable, the guide may also be useful in posterior areas with wide edentulous ridges.

- Such templates even more accurately locate the placement of an implant and direct the inclination of its long axis.
- Surgical templates can also be fabricated for a maxillary edentulous arch that is to be restored with a fixed prosthesis.

Q.151. A gnathodynameter is used to record:

1. Biting force
2. Centric relation
3. Vertical dimensions
4. FH plane

Ans. (1). Biting force *(Hertwell 4th ed., P. 535; Jablonski dictionary, Nallaswamy 1st ed., P. 783).*

Gnathodynamometer:

1. An instrument for measuring the force exerted in closing the jaws.
2. An instrument used for measuring biting pressure.

Q.152. For a patient with missing cauine what type of broshtesis we will prefer:

1. Three unit FPD
2. Resin retained FPD
3. Implant retained crown
4. It will depend on patient choice.

Ans. (3).Implant retained crown *(Rosenstiel 3rd ed., P. 65; Nallaswamy 1st ed., P. 525, Misch 3rd ed., P. 197).*

In case of a single missing canine, where a cantilever FPD is planned, support should be taken from both central and lateral incisor. It should also be remembered that the replacement of single missing maxillary canine is considered as a complex fixed partial denture because the tooth lies out side the interabutment axis and the adjacent teeth like the lateral incisor and the first premolar are very weak. This FPD will be subjected to forces acting in an outward direction.

(Nallaswamy 1st ed.)

A fixed prosthesis is not indicated if a canine and more than one adjacent tooth are missing so implant retained crown is best choice.

(Misch 3rd ed.)

More about implant supported fixed partial denture:

It is indicated in:

1. Absence of sufficient number of abutments for a long edentulous span.
2. Absence of distal abutment but presence of good density of bone.
3. Broad flat ridge configurations.

4. Single tooth replacements.
5. High carries risk patients.
6. Young adults
7. Inability to wear removable partial or complete denture.

Contraindication:

1. Acute illness
2. Terminal illness
3. Pregnancy
4. Uncontrolled metabolic disease
5. Tumoricidal radiation to the implant site
6. Unrealistic patient expectation
7. Improper patient motivation
8. Lack of operator experience
9. Inability to restore with prosthesis

Q.153. Ideal site for implant placement in a completely edeutulous mandible:

1. 1st molar region bilaterally
2. Retromolar pad area because it is resistant to resorption
3. Buccal shelf area because it is most ideally suited for loading.
4. Interforaminal region.

Ans. (4). Interforaminal region *(Rosenstiel 3rd ed., P. 319, 320; Misch 3rd ed., P. 226).*

Implant Location:

Anterior mandible:

Anterior mandible has adequate height and width for implant placement and the bone quality is normally excellent, which makes it require the least amount of time for integration. Implant should be placed in cancellous bone. The mental nerve is 3.0 mm anterior to the mental foramen before turning posteriorly and superiorly to exit at the foramen, it is recommended that an implant be at least 5 mm anterior to foramen i.e. interforaminal region.

Anterior maxilla:

The anterior maxilla must be evaluated for proximity to the nasal cavity. A minimum of 1 mm of bone should remain between the apex of the implant and the nasal vestibule.

Anterior maxillary implants should be located slightly off midline, on either side of the incisive foramen.

Posterior mandible:

The inferior alveolar nerve traverses the mandibular body in this region and the treatment planning must allow for a 20 mm margin from the apex of the implant to the superior aspect of the inferior alveolar canal. Implant placed in the posterior mandible are usually shorter, do not engage cortical bone inferiorly, and must support increased biomechanical occlusal forces once they are loaded.

Posterior maxilla:

Posterior maxilla has less dense bone, larger marrow space and thinner cortex. In treatment planning for implants in the posterior maxilla, the surgeon should leave 1 mm of bone between the floor of sinus and the implant so the implant can be anchored apically into cortical bone of sinus floor. Also see this topic from "Babush" Implantology.

Q.154. A patient with glaucoma should not receive:

1. Sedative
2. Vasoconstrictors
3. Antisialogues
4. Local anaesthetics

Ans. (3). Antisialogues *(Nallaswamy 1st ed., P. 623).*

Antisialogogues: These are group of drugs that can be effectively used to control salivary flow. They are gastro-intestinal anticholinergic that inhibit the action of myoepithelial cells in the salivary gland producing dry mouth.

Commonly used antisialogogues:

1. Methantheline bromide (Banthine) : 50 mg/hr before procedure.
2. Propantheline bromide (Pro-banthine) : 15 mg/hr before procedure.
3. Clonidine hydrochloride (Antihyper-tensive) : 0.2 mg/hr before procedure.
4. Atropine

Contraindications: Hypersensitive patients, patient with glaucoma, asthma, obstructive conditions of congestive heart failure etc.

(Nallaswamy)

Atrophic drugs (Antisialogogues) drug are absolutely contraindicated in individuals with a narrow iridocorneal angle may precipitate acute congestive glaucoma. However marked rise in intraocular tension is rare in patients with wide angle glaucoma.

Caution is advocated in elderly males with prostatic hypertrophy - urinary retention can occur.

(KDT)

Q.155. Pontic design not indicated in anterior region:

1. Ovate pontic
2. Modified ridge lap pontic
3. Stein pontic
4. Spheroidal pontic

Ans. (4). Spheroidal pontic *(Tylmann P. 357; Nallaswamy 1st ed., P. 571).*

Spheroidal and modified spheroidal pontic:

These pontics are used in mandibular posterior region.

(Tylmann)

Spheroidal and modified spheroidal pontics:

1. These pontics contact the tissue only at the ridgecrest.
2. These do not have contact gingival surfaces.
3. They are indicated for cases with reduced interarch space, where the pontic should give the appearance of an exaggerated occlusogingival dimension.

Saddle pontic: A pontic with a concave gingival surface that overlaps the ridge buccally and lingually is called a saddle. The gingival surface of the saddle pontic will not have continuous contact with the ridge instead only the buccal and lingual ends of the gingival surface will contact the tissue. These pontics are generally avoided because they are very difficult to maintain and it is impossible to avoid accumulation of food debris.

Sanitary or hygienic pontic: Sanitary pontic allows easy cleaning because its tissue surface remains clear of the residual ridge these pontics have zero tissue contact. Though they are easy to maintain, they are highly unaesthetic hence they are used only for posterior teeth. The pontic should be at least 3 mm high occlusogingivally and at same time provide adequate tissue clearance for easy maintenance.

Bullet shaped or conical or heart shaped pontic: This pontic has a convex tissue surface, which contact the tissue at one single point without any pressure. This pontic is very easy to clean and maintain. The only disadvantage of this design is its poor aesthetics, which results due to wide embrasures. It is indicated for the replacement of mandibular posterior teeth where aesthetics in not a major concern.

Ovate pontic: These pontics are used in cases where the residual ridge is defective or incompletely healed. They can also be used in broad and flat ridges. The pontic is designed such that its cervical end extends in to the defect of the residual ridge. The pontics should be reduced as healing progress. This pontic is more aesthetic as it appears to arise from the ridge like a natural tooth. It is said evolved from root extended or root tipped pontic.

Bullet shaped or conical or heart shaped pontic: This pontic has a convex tissue surface, which contact the tissue at one single point without any pressure. This pontic is very easy to clean and maintain. The only disadvantage of this design is its poor aesthetics, which result due to wide embrasures. It is indicated for the replacement of mandibular posterior teeth where aesthetics is not a major concern.

Ridge lap pontics : This pontic resemble a natural tooth. It is designed to adapt closely to the ridge. It is avoided because it is difficult to maintain and often leads to inflammation of the tissues in contact.

Modified ridge lap pontics : Ridge lap pontics evolved from saddle pontics. Though the ridge lap pontics had relatively less tissue contact, they were also difficult to maintain. Hence the ridge lap pontics were modified and evolved as the modified ridge lap pontics. Modified ridge lap pontics were designed to reduce the tissue contact. Generally this pontic is avoided because the buccolingual concavity is difficult to clean and maintain when the modified ridge lap pontic is further reduced, they are known as lap facings.

Q.156. Cavosurface margin angulation in chamfer finish line is:

1. Always 90°
2. 90° or less than 90°
3. 90° or more than 90°
4. 120°

Ans. (3).90° or more than 90° *(Rosenstiel 3rd ed., P. 175, 198, 226).*

Chamfer:

1. A finish line design for tooth preparation in which the gingival aspect meets the external axial surface at an obtuse angle (more than 90°).
2. A small groove or furrow.
3. The surface found by cutting away the angle of intersection of two faces of a piece of material (i.e. stone, metal, wood) a beveled edge.

Advantages:

- Distinct margin
- Adequate bulk
- Easier to control

Disadvantage:

Care needed to avoid unsupported lip of enamel.

Indications:

- Cast metal restoration
- Lingual margin of metal-ceramic crowns.

Q.157. In case, if maxillary canine is missing and we have to make a tooth supported FPD, abutments will be:

1. Central incisor, lateral incisor and 1st premolar
2. Lateral incisor, 1st premolar and 2nd premolar
3. Lateral incisor and 1st premolar
4. Ist depends upon periodontal status of remaining teeth.

Ans. (4). 1st depends upon periodontal status of remaining teeth *(Rosenstiel 3rd ed., P. 71)*.

Selection of abutment also depend on periodontal status of tooth.

- If horizontal bone loss occur the periodontal support root surface area is reduced.
- When root length is exposed, the supporting area is lost.
- Successful fixed prostheses can be fabricated on teeth with severely reduced periodontal support provided the periodontal tissue have been returned to excellent health and long term maintenance has been assured.
- Healthy periodontal tissue are a prerequisite for all fixed restorations.
- If the abutment teeth have normal bone support an occasional lapse in plaque removal by the patient is unlikely to affect the long term prognosis.
- When teeth with severe bone loss resulting from periodontal disease are used as abutments there is very little tolerance. It has become imperative that excellent plaque removal technique be implanted and maintained at all times.

So abutment selection depend on periodontal status.

Q.158. Training groove is placed in the lower denture:

1. To train the patients tongue position.
2. In case of mandibulectomy.
3. To train the orbicularis oris muscle
4. To train tognetic patient.

Ans. (1). Impression for complete denture by *Bernald Levine P. 58.*

- Many patients with a retruded tongue have an awkward tongue as well as they tend to have difficulties in placing and maintaing the correct tongue position.
- Training grooves of about 10 mm long 2 mm wide and 2 mm deep is made below the anterior central incisors in mandibular dentures and later on filled with auto-polymerising acrylic resin.
- This training groove is made to guide the normal tongue position.

Q.159. Pivoting movement better resisted by a tooth preparation if:

1. Diameter is smaller
2. Diameter is large
3. Diameter is large and length is small.
4. Do not depend on diameter of tooth.

Ans. (1). Diameter is smaller *(Schillinberg 3rd ed., P. 123).*

A preparation on a tooth with a smaller diameter resists pivoting movement better than a preparation of equal length on a tooth of large diameter.

Q.160. Shunting effect occurs in complete dentures:

1. If occlusal plane is lower in molar area.
2. If occlusal plane is lower in incisor area.
3. If occlusal plane is lower in molar as well incisor area.
4. When patient has poor muscular coordination.

Ans. (1). If occlusal plane is lower in molar area *(Impression for Complete Denture by Bernald Levine P. 27).*

- If occlusal plane is tipped, there will be a shunting effect and loss of stability.
- If the occlusal plane is longer in molar area there will be a tendency for the upper denture to be displaced posteriorly and the lower denture anteriorly.
- If occlusal plane is lower in incisor area, the shunting effect will be opposite to that given above.

Q.161. Malocclusion characterized by retroclined central and proclined lateral incisor is:

1. Class II Division I
2. Class II Division II
3. Class III
4. Class I

Ans. (2). Class II Division II *(Bhalajhi 2nd ed., P. 78, Rani 3rd ed., P. 21).*

Class II malocclusion: This group is characterized by a class II molar relation where distobuccal cusp of upper 1st permanent molar occludes in the buccal groove of lower 1st permanent molar.

Classification of Class II malocclusion:

Class II Division I : characterized by proclined upper incisors with a resultant increase in overjet.

Class II Division II : characterized by presence of lingually inclined upper central incisors and labially tipped upper lateral incisors overlapping the central incisors. Variation of this form are lingually inclined central and lateral incisor with the canine labially tipped.

Class II subdivison: When a class II molar relation exists on one side and class I relation on the other, it is referred to as class II subdivision.

Class II division I subdivision

Class II division II subdivision

Feature of class II division I:

Extraoral:

1. Convex profile
2. Short upper lip

3. Incompetent lips
4. Everted lower lip
5. Deep mentolabial sulcus
6. Hyperactive mentalis

Intraoral:

1. Class II molar relation (Distoocclusion)
2. Class II canine relation
3. Class II division I incisors
4. Deep bite
5. Crowding or spacing of teeth
6. Deep curve of spee
7. V shaped arch form
8. Deep palate

<u>Feature of class II division II:</u>

Extraoral:

1. Straight profile/mild convexity
2. Competent lips

Intraoral:

1. Class II molar relation
2. Class II canine relation
3. Class II division II incisor relation
4. Central incisors are retroclined
5. Lateral incisors are proclined and overlap the centrals
6. Occasionally central and lateral incisors are retroclined and canine are placed buccally
7. Overjet is decreased
8. Closed bite is present upper incisors are retroclined and overlap the lower incisors.
9. Deep curve of spee.
10. Broad and U shaped arch
11. Sometimes buccal crossbite is present.

Q.162. Which of the following forces best accomplish orthodontic tooth movement?

1. Heavy and continuous
2. Heavy and intermittent
3. Light and continuous
4. Light and intermittent

Ans. (3). Light and continuous *(Rani 3rd ed., P. 218, 220).*

Use of continuous light force is recommended to be applied for adult group of patients rather than intermittent force as applied by removable appliances. There is a need of continuous force to stimulate constant development of osteoclast in adults.

Various types of forces are:

Continuous force: Continuous force is generated by means of springs or elastic bands. Force should be limited to 20-26 gms per sq. cm of root surface area.

Interrupted type: This interrupted type is usually of shorter duration when compared to continuous tooth movement e.g.

1. Ligation of a lingually placed tooth to the labial arch.
2. In case of alignment of impacted canine.
3. Correction of open bite.

Intermittent force: Typical intermittent action is produced by a force that acts either as an impulse or as a shock of short duration with a series of interruption. It is an orthodontic or orthopedic force that is inactive for intervals of time between appointments.

Q.163. Relative to primary mandibular incisors, permanent mandibular incisors erupt:

1. Lingually
2. Facially
3. Distally
4. Mesially

Ans. (1). Lingually *(Bhalajhi 2nd ed., P. 57).*

The permanent dentition forms within the jaw soon after birth except for the cusp of 1st permanent molars which form before birth. The permanent incisors develop lingual or palatal to the deciduous incisors and move labially as they erupt.

This is one of the self correcting anomalies and should not be corrected unless it persist after 8 year of age. The tongue has a forward thrust on there teeth which bring these teeth to move labially and bring about the correction.

- Incisor erupt lingually.
- Canine erupt buccally.
- Premolar erupt palatally.
- Molar erupt buccally.

Q.164. In cephalometrics, the Frankfort plane is constructed:

1. Horizontally from nasion through porion.
2. Horizontally from nasion to the superior aspect of external auditory meatus.
3. Vertically from orbitale through the maxillary canine.
4. Horizontally from orbitale to the superior aspect of external auditory meatus.

Ans. (4). Horizontally from orbitale to the superior aspect of external auditory meatus *(Rani 3rd ed., P. 145, Bhalajhi 2nd ed., P. 150).*

Frankfurt Horizontal Plane (FH Plane):

The plane is drawn from Porion to orbitale. This plane was selected for the orientation of the skulls of different individual or of different species because it was thought that this plane approximate the true horizontal plane when an individual holds his head in normal relaxed natural position.

Importance of FH plane:

FH plane is useful in orienting the photographs or the study cast to the radiographs because it can be located on radiograph and even be usualized clinically.

Q.165. Six keys to normal occlusion were given by:

1. Andrews
2. Angle
3. Tweed
4. Steiner

Ans. (1). Andrews *(Bhalajhi 2nd ed., P. 70, Rani 3rd ed., P. 10).*

Six keys to normalocclusion were given by Lawrence F. Andrews. Andrews considered the presence of these feature essential to achieve an optimal occlusion. The six keys to normal occlusion are considered under the following headings.

1. **Molar interarch relationship:** The mesiobuccal cusp of upper first molar should occlude in groove between the mesial and medial buccal cusp of lower first molar.
2. **Mesidistal crown angulation:** Gingival part of long axis of crown must be distal to the occlusal part.
3. **Labiolingual crown inclination:** The maxillary incisor exhibit a positive crown inclination while mandibular incisor show mild negative crown inclination. The maxillary and mandibular posterior have negative crown inclination.
4. **Absence of rotation:** Normal occlusion is characterized by absence of any retation.
5. **Tight contact:** These should be tight contact between adjacent teeth.
6. **Curve of spee:** The curve of spee not exceeding 1.5 mm.

The seventh key to normal occlusion is Bolton ratio as asked in AIPG 2004.

Q.166. The permanent anterior tooth that most often shows variation in size is the:

1. Mandibular canine.
2. Mandibular central incisor.
3. Maxillary canine
4. Maxillary lateral incisor

Ans. (4). Maxillary lateral incisor *(Shafer 4th ed., P. 38).*

Microdontia involving a single tooth is a rather common condition. It affects most often the maxillary lateral incisor and the third molar.

Localised microdontia which affect the maxillary lateral incisor, a condition that has been called the "Peg lateral". Instead of exhibiting parallel or diverging mesial and distal surfaces the side coverage or taper together incisally forming a peg shaped or cone shaped crown. The root on such a tooth is frequently shorter than usual.

Q.167. Oral Screen:

1. Cause the child to breathe through the nose.
2. Allow for the passage of air through mouth.
3. Prevents passage of air through nares.
4. Allow the passage of air through mouth and nose.

Ans. (1). Cause the child to breathe through the nose *(Rani 3rd ed., P. 312, Bhalajhi 2nd ed., P. 323).*

Oral screen: Oral screen was first introduced by Newell in 1912.

Principle: The oral screen can be used either to apply the force of the circumoral musculature to certain teeth or to relieve those forces from the teeth thereby allowing them to move due to force exerted by tongue. This vestibular screen works on principle of both force application and force elimination. It is fitted in vestibule of mouth.

Indication: Oral screen is indicated for the correction of the following situation:

1. Mouth breathing
2. Thumb sucking
3. Lip biting
4. Tongue thrust
5. Mild distoocclusion with premaxillary protrusion and open bite in deciduous and mixed dentition.
6. In the presence of flaccid, hypotonic, orofacial musculature as muscle exerciser.
7. For the correction of proclined upper anterior teeth.

Modification of oral screen:

1. Oral screen with breathing holes.
2. Oral screen with embedded metal ring to be used as muscle exerciser.
3. Double oral screen for tongue thrusting and mouth breathing patients.
4. Hotz modification
5. Modification of Rehak
6. Polyamide or thermoplastic sheets for use in orthodontics.

Mechanism of Action:

1. It acts like a mechanical barrier and helps in correction of some oral habits.
2. In presence of proclination of upper anterior teeth the oral screen is designed to contact only those teeth. When the patient close the lips or swallows, all the muscle force are transmitted to anterior teeth. There is no counter acting force for tongue on the buccal aspect of posterior teeth. This result in buccal movement of posterior teeth or expansion of arches.
3. When used as muscle exerciser the hypotonic muscles are induced to work.

(Rani 3rd ed.)

Most effective way to reestablish nasal breathing is to prevent air from entering the oral cavity and for this lip or oral cavity are closed.

(Shobha Tandon 1st ed.)

Q.168. Which of the following is the least stable orthodontic correction:

1. Maxillary expansion
2. Rotations
3. Overbite
4. Overjet

Ans. (2). Rotations *(Rani 3rd ed., P. 216; Bhalajhi 2nd ed., P. 380).*

Rotation: It is the movement of the tooth around the long axis. It is a difficult type of tooth movement to correct and retain. Rotations are best effected by dissipating force with period of stabilizations. Correction of rotation require couple force. High relapse tendencies with rotation is because of presence of elastic fibres in supra alveolar tissues. Over correction of transaction or supra alveolar fibres might be of help in reducing the relapse tendencies. These gingival group of fibres takes as much as 232 days of even longer for recognisation.

Q.169. According to Wolff's law:

1. Human teeth drift mesially as interproximal wear occurs.
2. Pressure cause bone resorption
3. Optimum level of force for moving teeth is 10-200 grams.
4. Bone trabeculae line up in response to mechanical stresses.

Ans. (4). Bone trabeculae line up in response to mechanical stresses *(Bhalajhi 2nd ed., P. 64; Rani 3rd ed., P. 218).*

Wolf's Law of Transformation of Bone:

Bone elements once formed rearrange themselves in the direction of functional pressure and increase and decrease their mass to reflect the functional stress.

(Rani 3rd ed.)

Bone unlike other connective tissue responds to mild degree of pressure and tension by changes in its form.

This may take place on the surface of the bone under the periosteion or in the case of cancellous bone on the surface of trabeculae or an the walls of marrow spaces or air sinuses. The architecture of a bone is such that it can best resist the forces which are brought to bear upon it with the use of a little tissue as possible. It has been found that bone is formed in just the quality and shape that will enable it to withstand the physical demands made upon it with the greatest amount of economy of structure. This is the basis of Wolff's law of transformation of bone.

(Bhalajhi 2nd ed.)

Q.170. Resistance units of equal size pulling against each is an example of which form of anchorage:

1. Cortical anchorage
2. Reciprocal anchorage
3. Reinforced anchorage
4. Stationary anchorage.

Ans. (2).Reciprocal anchorage *(Rani 3rd ed., 227; Bhalajhi 2nd ed., P. 212).*

Classification of anchorage (Moyers):

According to the manner of force application:

1. Simple anchorage
2. Stationary anchorage
3. Reciprocal anchorage

According to jaw involved:

1. Intermaxillary
2. Intramaxillary

According to the site of anchorage:

1. Intra oral
2. Extra oral
   - Cervical
   - Occipital
   - Cranial
   - Facial
3. Muscular

According to number of anchorage unit:

1. Single or primary anchorage
2. Compound anchorage
3. Multiple or reinforced anchorage

Reciprocal anchorage: The term refers to the resistance offered by two malposed units when the dissipation of equal and opposite forces tend to move each unit towards a more normal occlusion e.g.

1. Reciprocal anchorage include closure of midline diastema by moving two central incisor towards each other.
2. Use of cross bite elastics.
3. Dental arch expansion.

Q.171. Single force applied at which point of a tooth will allow complete translation of the tooth:

1. At the apex
2. At the incisal edge.
3. At the center of resistance.
4. At the center of rotation.

Ans. (3). At the center of resistance *(Rani 3rd ed., P. 214-215, Bhalajhi 2nd ed., P. 204).*

When the line of action of force passes through center of resistance the tooth will be translated in the direction of force vector. If the line of action of force does not pass through the center of resistance it result in tipping of tooth. If the force does not pass through the long axis of the tooth it result in rotation.

Translation or bodily tooth movement:

By the use of couple or application of force at more than one point on the surface of a tooth, bodily tooth movement can be accomplished.

Tissue reaction: When a lingual moving force is applied, resorption along the entire lingual surface of the alveolus occurs. Bone apposition take place along the entire labial surface. Bodily tooth movement is the ideal type of tooth movement and is preferable to the tipping movement. However root resorption is observed more frequently with this type of tooth movement and hence the force used to move the tooth should not exceed limits.

Translation is brought about by an appropriate combination of force and couple.

Force required:

- Small teeth - 40-50 gms.
- Large teeth - 150 gms.

Q.172. Which of the fibres attached to cementum are most likely to contribute to relapse of tooth rotation?

1. Apical fibres.
2. Gingival group of fibres.
3. Horizontal fibres.
4. Oblique fibres.

Ans. (2). Gingival group of fibres *(Rani 3rd ed., P. 216, 236; Bhalajhi 2nd ed., P. 380).*

- High relapse tendencies with rotation is because of presence of elastic fibres in supra alveolar tissue.
- Tension produced by transeptal fibres or gingival connective tissue fibres that have not been removed during tooth movement.
- Pericision or circumferential supracrestal fibrotomy is an adjunctive surgical procedure where the gingival fibres are incised to prevent relapse. If it is done after orthodontic treatment helps in retention of corrected rotated position of the tooth.

Q.173. Which is the predominant factor in the formation of alveolar process:

1. Eruption of teeth.
2. Normal process of growth.
3. Lengthening of the Condyle.
4. Overall growth of the bodies of the maxilla and the mandible.

Ans. (1). Eruption of teeth *(Bhalajhi 2nd ed., P. 41).*

- The alveolar process develops in response to the presence of tooth buds. As the teeth erupt, the alveolar process develops and increase in height by bone deposition at the margins.
- The alveolar bone adds to the height and thickness of the body of the mandible and is particularly manifested as a ledge extending lingual to the ramus to accommodate the 3rd molars.
- In case of absence of teeth, the alveolar bone fails to develop and it resorbs in the event of tooth extraction.

Q.174. The last primary tooth to be replaced by a permanent tooth is usually:

1. Maxillary canine.
2. Mandibular canine
3. Maxillary first molar
4. Mandibular second molar

Ans. (1). Maxillary canine *(Profitt 3rd ed., P. 85, 86).*

- At deutal age 11, the only remaining primary teeth are the maxillary canine, second molar and mandibular second molar.
- At deutal age 12, the remaining succedaneous maxillary canine permanent teeth erupt. Succedaneous refers to permanent teeth that replace primary predecessors, thus a maxillary canine is a succedaneous tooth here - Profitt P. 85.
- Labial positioning of maxillary canine often occurs when there is an overall lack of space in the arch, because this is the last tooth to erupt normally.

(Profitt P. 86)

Q.175. The midpalatal suture is most likely to open at which following ages of expansion?

1. 18 years old
2. 13 years old
3. 25 years old
4. 55 years old

Ans. (2).13 years old *(Profitt 3rd ed., P. 534).*

- It is relatively easy to widen the maxilla by opening the mid palatal suture before and during adolescence, but this become progressively more difficult as the patient become older.
- The chances of successful opening of the suture are nearly 100% before the age 15, but begin to decline thereafter because of the increased interdigitation of the suture.
- So the opening of mid palatal suture should be done before 15 years of age so the answer is 13 years.

Note:

1. Ossification of the palate occur from 8th week of intrauterine life.
2. This is an intra-membranous type of ossification
3. The mid palatal suture ossifies by 12-14 years.

Q.176. Functional appliances:

1. Only move teeth
2. Can change the direction of growth.
3. Are fabricated in the original mandibular position.
4. Correct malocclusion rapidly.

Ans. (2). Can change the direction of growth *(Rani 3rd ed., P. 309; Bhalajhi 2nd ed., P. 315).*

Functional Appliance: or myofunctional applicances as they are sometimes referred to are appliance that depend upon the orofacial musculature for their action.

- The force component of functional applicances are derived from the orofacial musculature. These appliance either transmit, eliminate or guide the natural force of the musculature.
- Functional appliances are used for growth modification procedure that are aimed at intercepting and treating jaw discrepancies. They can bring about the following changes.

1. An increase or decrease in jaw size.
2. A change in spatial relationship of the jaws.
3. Change in direction of growth of the jaws.
4. Acceleration of desirable growth.

Functional appliances are defined as loose fitting or passive appliances which harness natural forces or orofacial musculature that are transmitted to the teeth and alveolar bone through the medium of the appliance.

Limitations of functional appliances:

1. They can be used to correct basal bone/arch relationship and can not be used for correcting dental malocclusion.

2. It is not useful in managing adult patients where the active growth is completed.
3. It require a final phase of fixed appliance therapy to achieve final detailing or final alignment of tooth position.
4. The result of treatment is totally dependent upon the patients cooperation.
5. They have a tendency to increase the lower facial height and hence they cannot be used in patients with back-ward rotating mandible.

Q.177. The tactile threshold of the natural teeth during axial loading:

1. .001-.01 N
2. 0.01-0.10 N
3. 0.10-0.50 N
4. 1-2 N

Ans. (2).0.01-0.10 N. Management of temporomandibular disorder and occlusion by *Jeffery Okeson 5th ed., P. 49, 119, 120; Journals of Prosthetic Dentistary Jan. 2004 P. 31*

Axial loading: The process of directing occlusal forces through the long axis of the tooth is known as axial loading. Axial loading can be achieved by two methods.

1. First method is through development of tooth contacts on either cusptips or relatively flat surfaces that are perpendicular to the long axis of the tooth. These flat surfaces canbe the crest of marginal ridges or the bottoms of fossal with this type of contact the resultant forces will be directed through the long axis of the tooth.
2. The second method of axial loading called tripodization requires that each cusp contacting on opposing fossa be developed such that it produces three contacts surrounding the actual cusp tip. When this is achieved the resultant force is directed through the long axis of the tooth.

Both methods eliminate off axis forces, thereby allowing the PDL to accept effectively potentially damaging forces to the tone and essentially reduce them.

Force of mastication: the maximum biting force that canbe applied to the teeth varies from individual to individual. It is generally found that males can bite with more force than can female. Female's maximum biting load ranges from 79-99 pounds (35.8-44.9 kg) while a male biting load varies from 118-142 pounds (53.6-64.4 kg). The greatest maximum biting force reported in 975 pounds (443 kg). It has also been noted that the maximum amount of force applied to a molar is usually several times that which can be applied to an incisor.

Range of maximum force applied to first molar was 91-198 (41.3-89.8 kg) where as the maximum force applied to central incisor was 29-51 pound (13.2-23.1 kg). The maximum biting force appear to increase with age up to adolescent.

Note: During each chewing stroke an average of 58.7 pounds of force is applied to the teeth for 115 msec.

- Force of tooth contact for functional activity is 17200Lb/sec/day.
- Force of tooth contact for para-functional activity is 57600 Lb/sec/day.
- Intra oral load (force) vary from 10-43 IN (IN = 0.225 Lb of force).
- Functional load of 70 N of considered normal.
- According to Sturdevent, during mastication pressure exerted on teeth is 150-500 pound.

(Jeffery Okeson)

The mean value for threshold for tactile perception of ITI dental implants ranged from 13.2–189.4

gm (0.132–1.894 N) while for natural teeth it ranged from 1.2–26.2 g (0.012–0.262 N)

Tactile sensation threshold for ITI dental implant in edentulous subject varied from 148–1300 gm (1.48–13 N) in vertical direction where as in horizontal direction the force varied from 118–200 gm (1.18 to 12 N).

(Journals of Prothetic Dentistary)

Q.178. Which position is most important in diagnosis of anterior or posterior cross bite?

1. Habitual position.
2. Lateral shift.
3. Maximum interucspation
4. The point of first contact at centric relation.

Ans. (4). The point of first contact at centric relation *(Shobha Tondon 1st ed., P. 413)*.

Anterior cross bite:

Etiology:

1. Traumatic injury to the primary dentition that cause a lingual displacement of the permanent bud.
2. Supernumerary tooth.
3. A habit of biting the upper lip.
4. A repaired cleft lip
5. Anterior cross bite of skeletal origin generally results from on excessive abnormal mandibular growth that produce a true class III malocclusion.

Posterior cross bite:

Etiology:

1. Ectopic eruption of the permanent first molar.
2. Prolonged thumb or finger sucking.
3. Prolonged retention of primary teeth.
4. Occlusal interference.
5. Skeletal - They may be caused due to:
   - Deficient lateral growth of the maxilla as seen in cleft palate repair.
   - Increased growth of mandible or

- Combination of both

Diagnosis of anterior cross bite is made by a functional cross bite caused due to premature tooth contact during centric closure.

Diagnosis of posterior cross bite made by occlusal interference which cause functional shift of mandible to a maximum interauspation.

Q.179. Reduced salivary flow following irradiation is dose dependent. At what dose does the flow reach essentially zero.

1. 4000 rads
2. 5000 rads
3. 6000 rads
4. 7000 rads

Ans. (3).6000 rads *(White and Pharoah 4th ed., P. 30).*

The parenchymal component of the salivary gland is radio sensitive. The first few weeks after initiation of radiotherapy usually sees a marked and progressive loss of salivary secretion. The extent of reduced flow is dose dependent and reaches essentially zero at 60 Gy (6000 rads). The mouth become dry (xerostomia) and tender and swallowing is difficult and painful because the residual saliva also loses its normal lubricating properties.

(White 4th ed.)

Read text below:

Critical organ	Risk or threshold dose
Skin (Cancer)	25000 mrad
Red bone marrow (Leukemia)	5000 mrad
Eye (Cataracts)	200000 mrad
Thyroid (Cancer)	6500 mrad
Breast (Cancer)	No threshold
Gonads (Mutation, infertility, Fetal malformations)	No threshold
Taste buds	1000-10000 rads
Salivary gland	6000 rads

Q.180. Which of the following is used to show the base of skull spheroid sinus, position and orientation of Condyles and fractures of the zygomatic arch?

1. The TMJ surgery
2. Submentovertex projection
3. Reverse Towne projection
4. The facial profile survey

Ans. (2). Submentovertex projection *(White and Pharoah 4th ed., P. 201, 202).*

The submentovertex projection (also called the base or full axial projection is used to demonstrate the base of skull the position and orientation of the condyles, the sphenoid sinus, the curvature of mandible, the lateral wall of the maxillary sinuses and any displacement of a fractured sygomatic arch. Often this view also displays the medial and lateral pterygoid plates and foramina in the base of skull.

Film placement: The film cassette is placed vertically in a holding device.

Head position: The patient's head and neck should be entended backward as far as possible with the vertex of the skull on the center of the cassette. However the midsaggital plane of the head must remain perpendicular to the floor. The cantomeatal line should extend 10 degree past vertical so that the Frankfort line is vertical and parallel to film.

Projection of the central rays: The central says is directed from below the mandible upward toward the vertex of the skull, and is positioned far enough anterior to pass about 2 cm in front of a line connecting the right and left condylar processes.

Exposure parameters: When a film and screen combination with a speed class of 250 is used with a KVP of 70, the mAs should be about 100. For viewing the zygomatic arches especially the exposure time is reduced to one third that used to visualize the skull.

Read text below:

Maxillary sinus	⟶	Water's view
Zygoma fracture	⟶	Occipito mental view
Base of skull	⟶	Submentovertex, Towne's projection
Nasal septum	⟶	Occipitomental view
Coronoid process of mandible	⟶	PA view of skull
Condylar neck fracture	⟶	Reverse Towne view
Zygomatic arch fracture	⟶	Submentovertex
Fracture of ramus and body of mandible	⟶	Lateral oblique 15°
Medially displaced fracture of condyle	⟶	PA view
Horizontal favourable and unfavourable fracture of mandible	⟶	Lateral oblique 30°
Midmandibular ramus to condylar apex	⟶	Transpharyngeal view

Q.181. Which survey has the purpose of examining fracture of condylar neck of the mandible?

1. Lateral jaw projection
2. Lateral skull projection
3. Waters projection
4. Reverse-Townes view

Ans. (4). Reverse-Townes view *(White and Pharoah 4th ed., P. 198, 201).*

Reverse-Towne's projection is used to examine radiographically a patient suspected of having a condylar fracture of neck. This projection is particularly suitable for revealing a medially displaced condyle. The Reverse-Towne's projection also reveals the posterolateral wall of the maxillary antrum.

Film placement: The cassette is positioned in a holding device.

Head position: The head should be centered in front of the cassette with the canthomeatal line oriented downward 25-30°. The condyles are better visualized if the patient opens the mouth as wide as possible.

Projection of central ray: The central ray is directed toward the film in the saggital plane through the occipital bone.

Exposure parameter: When a film and screen combination is used having a speed class of 250 with a KVP of 70, the mAs should be about 100.

Q.182. In Radionuclide imaging the most useful radio pharmaceutical for skeletal imaging is:

1. Gallium 67 (^{67}Ga)
2. Technetium-sulphur-colloid (^{99m}TC-SC)
3. Technetium-99m (^{99m}TC)
4. Technetium-99m linked to methylene disphosphonate (^{99m}TC-MDP)

Ans. (4). Technetium-99m linked to methylene disphosphonate (^{99m}TC-MDP) *(Harrison 15th ed., P. 1983).*

- ^{99m}TC lined to methylene diphosphonate or pertechnetate is most useful for bone imaging and useful in identifying.

1. Infection
2. Neoplasia
3. Inflammation
4. Increased blood flow
5. Bone remodeling
6. Heterotropic bone formation
7. Avascular necrosis

Read text below:

Scans	Used for
TC scan	Bone, liver, kidney, ventriculography
TC - albumin scan	Myocardial function
TC - pyrophosphate scan	In acute MI (hot spots)
TC - thallium substraction scan	Parathyroid gland
TC - labeled RBC	Spleen disease
Thallium scan	Myocardial perfusion
Gallium scan	Tumours
TC-SC scan	Reticuloendothelial system
Xenongas	Lung ventilation
Chromium	RBC
DTPA	GFR (Renal Excretory Function)
DMSA	Cortical function
Selenium^{75} methionin	Pancrease
Selenium and I^{131}	Thyroid
I^{131}, I^{132}	Placental function
I^{131} orthohippurate	Kidney

Q.183. The technique employed in radiotherapy to counteract the effect of tumour motion due to breathing is known as:

1. Arc technique
2. Modulation
3. Gating
4. Shunting

Ans. (4). Gating *(Walter and Miller 6th ed., P. 115).*

Gating is used inradiotherapy to counteract the effect of tumour motion due to breathing. In this technique 4 dimensional radiotherapy is used which gives radiation and move according to breathing cycle.

Shunting is technique like VP shunting to compress the tumour mass especially during pineal tumours.

Modulation is technique of intensity modulation to give radiotherapy to distally placed tumours.

Arc technique is a logical extension of multiple fixed technique is to have an infinite number of fields all aimed at one centre.

Q.184. Gamma camera in nuclear medicine is used for:

1. Organ imaging
2. Measuring the radioactivity
3. Monitoring the surface contamination
4. RIA

Ans. (1). Organ imaging *(Walter and Miller 6th ed., P. 112).*

- Gamma cameras are the devices used to observe the distribution of an isotope in an organ or in a part of the body.
- The multiple collimator is placed near the patient, a distribution of scintillation is produced in the crystal which corresponds to the distribution of isotope in field of view covered by the crystal and collimator.

Q.185. Ormocers are:

1. Organically modified composites
2. Inorganically modified composites
3. Organically modified glass ionomer cement.
4. Inorganically modified glass ionomer cement.

Ans. (1). Organically modified composites *(Vimal Sikri 1st ed., P. 413).*

Ormocers:

The omocers are organically modified ceramic can be used as a restorative material for both anterior and posterior teeth. Ormocers virtually replace amalgams and composites. Chemically it differs from composite in matrix constituents traditional composite are based on BISGMA, TEGDMA etc. Ormocer matrix consist of ceramic polysiloxane. The polysiloxane is biocompatible and exhibit low shrinkage. It contains 20-25% of matrix and rest is filler and coloring agents.

Physical properties:

Compressive strength - 420 mPa (62000 Psi)

Vicker Hardners - 80

Polymerisation shrinkage - 1.88%

Water sorption - 10.4 mg/mm^3

Fluoride release - positive

Advantage:

1. Biocompatible
2. Reduce polymerization shrinkage
3. High abrasion resistance, used in stress bearing area.

4. Esthetically pleasing
5. Anti-caries properties due to fluoride release
6. Safe handling, easy manipulation
7. Cost effective.

Q.186. Caries detection dye can stain the following except:

1. Granular necrotic tissue
2. Dry leathery dentin
3. Reversibly denatured collagen
4. Irrevesibly denatured collagen

Ans. (3). Reversibly denatured collagen
(Sturdevent 3rd ed., P. 296, 297).

Read text below:

Caries detection dye stain the infected dentin, granular necrotiç tissue, dry leatherydentin, irreversibly denatured collagen and not reversibly denatured collage.

Affected and infected dentin:

Affected dentin:

Affected dentin is reversibly denatured, not infected, remineralizable and should be preserved.

Infected dentin:

Bacteria is present in infected dentin. Infected dentin is softened. It include the superficial granular, necrotic tissue and softened, dry leathery dentin, irreversibly denatured (the collagen), not remineralizable and must be removed.

Dyes:

For detection of affected and infected dentin the dye 1% acid red 52 (acid rhodamine B or food red 106) in propylene glycol is used. This solution stain the outer layer (infected dentin), irreversibly denatured collagen in the outer carious layer but not the reversibly denatured collagen in the inner carious layer.

Basic fuschin dye was considered to be carcinogenic. Therefore it has been replaced by acid red and methylene blue. Methylene blue is also slightly toxic so acid red is preferred.

Other dyes are used for detection of carious enamel.

1. Procion dyes
2. Basic fuschin
3. Calcein dye
4. Fluoroscent dye (zyglo ZL-22)
5. Brilliant blue
6. Acid red
7. Methylene blue

Q.187. All of the following are true for traditional solution liner, except:

1. It is not necessary in moderately deep cavities under glass ionomer restoration.
2. Have film thickness of 1-50 microns.
3. Do not provide thermal or electric insulation.
4. Protect the pulp from reaction products leaching out of restoration.

Ans. (2). Have film thickness of 1-50 microns *(Sturdevent 3rd ed., P. 236, 240).*

- Liners are relatively thin layer of material used primarily to provide a barrier to protect the dentin from residual reactants, diffusing out of a restoration and/or oral fluid which may penetrate leaky tooth restoration interfaces. They also contribute initial electrical insulation generate some thermal protection, provide pulpal treatment as well.
- Thin film liners (1-50 μm) can be divided in to solution liners (varnishes, 2-5 μm) and suspension liners (typically 20-25 μm). Thicker liner (200-1000 μm), selected primarily for pulpal medication and thermal protection.
- For moderately deep cavity preparation, liners may be placed for thermal protection and pulpal medication.
- Any liner based on nonaqueous solvent evaporation for hardening is designated as a solution liner (or varnish).
- Liner based on water have many of the constituents suspended instead of dissolved and are called suspension liners.

- Solution liner have film thickness of 2-5 μm. A single coat effectively cover only 55% of the surface. A second thin layer is recommended to produce sealing of 80-85% of surface.

Solution liner (varnish):

Components: 10% copalresin, 90% ether, acetone, alcohol

Setting reaction: Physical

Solubility (% in water): Low

Tensile strength (mPa): <<1

Elongation (%): <<0.1% (Brittle)

Physical properties: Thermal and electrical insulator.

Q.188. One of the following is not true about treatment of dentinal hypersensitivity with dentin bonding agents:

1. It denatures protein
2. It forms a hybrid layer
3. It does not alter dentin permeability
4. It forms resin tags in to dentinal tubules.

Ans. (3). It does not alter dentin permeability *(Vimal Sikri 1st ed., P. 357).*

- Dentin bonding agent applied to dentin form hybrid layer, is best achieved by acidic conditioning agent which remove the smear layer, produce surface demineralization to a depth of 3-6 μms and expose the dentinal collagen framework.
- Conditioning of dentin cause alteration of dentin surface including the smear layer with the objective of producing a substrate capable of micromechanical and chemical bonding toa-dentin adhesive.
- Effect produced are the increase or decrease in the thickness and morphology of smear layer and also the dentinal tubules where as chemical effects are modification of the fraction of organic matter such as denaturation of proteins and decalcification of the inorganic portion.
- The major role of these agents is formation and stabilization of hybrid layer, production of resin tags in the unplugged dentinal tubules and at the same time sealing them to reduce the chance of increased permeability and thus pulpal irritation.
- When the adhesive resin is applied, a part of it

penetrates in to the microporous collagen scaffold of the inter tubular dentin known as intertubular penetration. Here it polymerize and copolymerize with the adhesion promotors of primers to form an intermingled layer hybrid layer, resin interdiffusion zone.

- The rest of the adhesive resin enters in to the dentinal tubules to a limited depth of 10-20 μms forming resin tags known as intratubular penetration.

Q.189. Amalgam achieves 70% of the strength by:

1. 2 hours
2. 4 hours
3. 8 hours
4. 16 hours

Ans. (3).8 hours *(Skinner 10th ed., P. 379).*

- Amalgam do not gain strength as rapidly as might be desired.
- At the end of 20 minute, the compressive strength may be only 6% of the 1 week strength.
- The ADA specification stipulates a minimum compressive strength of 80 mPa at one hour.
- The one hour compressive strength of high copper single composition amalgams is exceptionally high. This strength may have some advantages clinically e.g. fracture is less probable if the patient accidentally bites on the restoration soon after leaving the dental office. Also these amalgams may be strong enough shortly after placement to permit amalgams may be strong enough shortly after placement to permit amalgam build-ups to be prepared for crowns and to permit taking impressions for crowns.
- Even if a fast hardening amalgam is used, its strength is likely to be low initially. Patient should be cautioned not to subject the restoration to high biting stress for at least 8 hours after placement. By that time, a typical amalgam has reached at least 70% of its strength.
- Even at the end of a six month period some amalgams may still be increasing in strength.

Q.190. Torsional force is:

1. Compression
2. Tensile force
3. Shear
4. Transverse bending force

Ans. (3). Shear *(Skinner 11th ed., P. 78).*

Shear stress is produced by a twisting or torsional action on material.

Compressive stress: This type of stress tend to compress or shorten the material.

Tensile stress: Tends to strech or elongate a body.

Flexure (Bending stress): Produced by applied forces that causes flexural or torsional deformation.

Flexion is transverse bending force.

Q.191. Which of the following is not true about hand instruments used in operative dentistry?

1. They are generally made of stainless steel.
2. Nickel-cobalt-chromium is never used in its fabrication.
3. Carbon steel is more efficient than stainless steel.
4. It can be made with stainless steel with carbide inserts.

Ans. (2). Nickel-cobalt-chromium is never used in its fabrication *(Sturdevent 3rd ed., P. 326, Vimal Sikri 1st ed., P. 132).*

- Hand cutting instruments are manufactured from two main materials: carbon steels and stainless steel.
- Some hand cutting instruments are made with carbide inserts to provide more durable cutting edges.
- Carbon steel is harder than stainless steel, but when unprotected, it will corrode.
- Stainless steel remain bright under most conditions but loses a keen edge during use much more quickly than carbon steel.
- Carbide, while hard and wear resistant is brittle and cannot be used in all designs.
- Other alloy of nickel, cobalt, chromium are used in the manufacture of hand instruments but they are usually restricted to instruments other than those used for cutting of tooth structure.

(Sturdevent 3rd ed.,)

Carbon steel: It is an alloy made by addition

of small percentage of carbon to iron. It is capable of being hardened, softened and tempered. Its melting point is 1500°-1600° C.

There are two varieties of steel.

1. Soft steel
2. Hard steel.

Soft steel contains 0.5% or less of carbon while hard steel contains from 0.5-1.5% carbon. Other ingredient are manganese 0.2%, silicone 0.2% and the rest is iron (98.4-98.6%).

Stainless metals:

1. Stainless steel
2. Monel metal
3. Nichrome
4. Stellite
5. Tarno

(Vimal Sikri 1st ed.)

Q.192. Which of the following agent is used as a die hardner?

1. Cynoacrylate
2. Nail polish
3. Volatile relief agents.
4. Composite resin

Ans. (1). Cynoacrylate *(Vimal Sikri 1st ed., P. 267).*

Die Hardner:

- Certain water substitutes can dramatically increase the strength and hardness of gypsum e.g. aqueous solution of colloidal silica or soluble resin solution by increasing the friction between the dihydrate crystals.
- Gypsum products are modified to make the material more abrasion resistant. This can be done by using die hardening agent such as cyanoacrylate and acrylic resin lacquer.
- These hardening agents must be used in very thin coats to avoid any unacceptably thick relief at the margins of the preparation.
- The thickness of cyanoacrylates at the margin can range from 1.0-2.5 mm while acrylic lacquer can add to 4-10 mm thickness.

Die Spacer:

The most common die spacer are resins, models paints, coloured nail polish or thermoplastic polymers dissolved in volatile solvents may also be used. Usually a 20-40 mm is desired.

Q.193. Cavity formation in a tooth, due to dental caries is due to

1. Destructive potential of streptococcus mutAns.
2. Destructive potential of lactobacillus acidophilus
3. Lateral spread of caries along DE junction and weakening of overlying enamel.
4. Masticatory force and unrelated to the extent of carious process.

Ans. (3).Lateral spread of caries along DE junction and weakening of overlying enamel *(Sturdevent 3rd ed., P. 89; Vimal Sikri 1st ed., P. 22, 23).*

Read text below:

When the carious lesion has penetrated the enamel, it spread laterally along the dentinoenamle junction undermining the enamel. The lesion then invades dentin along the dentinal tubules. The pattern of invasion is depicted as cone shaped lesion with its base at the dentinoenamel junction and apex toward the pulp.

Histopathology of dentinal caries:

1. Zone of decomposed dentin
2. Zone of bacterial invasion
3. Zone of demineralization
4. Zone of dentinal sclerosis or hyper-mineralisation.
5. Zone of fatty degeneration
6. Zone of reparative dentin

(Vimal Sikri 1st ed.)

Q.194. Which of the following is not true about lubricant for rubber dam placement?

1. Should have water-miscible vehicle.
2. Vaseline is an ideal choice.
3. Should be easy to remove.
4. Should not interfere with bonding procedures.

Ans. (2). Vaseline is an ideal choice *(Gillmore 4th ed., P. 108).*

Lubricants:

Application of the rubber dam is simplified by the use of water soluble lubricant. They are placed on the tissue side of the rubber to fascilitate passing the material between the contact of tooth. Lubrication is advantageous when firm contact is defective and rough surfaces are in the isolated quadrant. The lubricant is placed only over the punched holes since these are the only areas of the rubber dam that pass between the teeth. Many solution have been advocated as lubricant. Most popular of these are soap, shaving cream and water soluble oil. All of these compounds are readily removed from enamel surface after the dam application in order to prevent contamination and adaptation problems for the restorative materials. Petroleum jelly (Vaseline) leaves a difficult to remove film and is not recommended.

Q.195. The range of wavelength of visible curing systems is:

1. 400-700 nm
2. 410-500 nm
3. 365-400 nm
4. 700-900 nm

Ans. **(2).**410-500 nm *(Sturdevent 3rd ed., P. 260).*

- Curing efficiency is strongly related to the effectiveness of light energy penetration in to the composite.
- Visible light curving involves light energy in the range of 410-500 nm with a peak intensity of about 470 nm.
- The intensity of light striking the composite depends on the output of the curing light itself and its distance from the composite.
- The intensity of light striking the composite is inversely proportional to the distance from the tip of fibrooptic bundle of the curing light to the dental composite surface.
- Ideally the tip should be with 2 mm of dental composite to the effective.
- The output energy should be about 300mW/cm^2 to be assured of adequate composite curing.

Q.196. Nanofillers are in the range of:

1. 10-100 microns
2. 0.1-1 microns
3. 0.01-0.1 microns
4. 0.005-0.01 microns

Ans. (4). 0.005-0.01 microns *(Sturdevent 3rd ed., P. 256).*

Classification of composite is based on the range of filler particle size. Composite filler particle are called mega fillers are in range of more than 100 microns. Microfillers are in the range of 10-100 mirons.

Midifillers from 1-10 microns.

Microfillers from 0.01-0.1 microns.

Ultra small filers (nanofillers) from 0.005-0.01 microns.

Composite with mixed range of particle size are called hybrids, and the largest particle size range is used to define the hybrid type (e.g. minifill hybrid)

If the composite simply consist of fillers and uncured matrix material it is classified as homogenous. If it includes precured composite or other unusual filler, it is called heterogenous. Precured particles were generated by grinding cured composite to a 1-20 micron size.

Q.197. Which one of the following does not commonly survive in a periapical lesion.

1. Pseudomonas
2. Streptococcus
3. Porphyromonas
4. Actinomyces

Ans. (1). Pseudomonas *(Ingle 4th ed., P. 615; Cohen Burns 8th ed., P. 503).*

Bacteria from periradicular tissue

Microorganisms	Percentage of anaerobes
Bacteroides	66%
Fusobacteriumnucleatum	48%
S. mitis, Grampositive facultative cocci, gram negative anaerobic rods	70%
Vellionella S. milleri	45% - strict 55% - Facultative
Eubacterium Propionibacterium	Not given
G +ve cocci G -ve cocci G +ve rods G -ve rods	65% - strict 28% - Facultative

(Ingle 4th ed.)

Bacteria from the root canals of teeth with apical rarefaction:

Bacteria	Percentage of incidences
Fusobacteriumnucleatum	48
Streptococcus sp.	40
Bacteroides sp.	35
Prevotella intermedia	34
Peptostreptococcus micros	34
Eubacterium alactolyticum	31
Peptostreptococcus anaerobius	32
Lactobacillus sp.	32
Eubacterium lectum	31
Fusobacterium sp.	29
Campylobacter sp.	25
Peptostreptococcus sp.	15
Actinomyces sp.	15
Eubacterium timidum	11
Capnocytophaga ochracea	11
Eubacterium brachy	9
Selenomonas sputigena	9
Vellionella parvula	9
Porphyromonas odontalis	9
Prevotella Buccal	9
Prevotella oris	8
Propniobacterium propniocum	8
Prevotella denticola	6
Prevotella loescheii	6
Eubacterium nodatum	6

(Cohen Burns 8th ed.)

Q.198. In Endodontic surgery, which of the following about chromic gut suture is not true:

1. Its properties are inferior to plain gut suture.
2. It is coated with chromium trionide.
3. It is less biocompatible than plain gut suture.
4. Its absorption is faster than plan gut suture.

Ans. (4). Its absorption is faster than plan gut suture *(Carranza 9th ed., P. 767).*

Read text below:

Nonabsorbable:

– Silk - braided.
– Nylon - monofilament (Ethilon)
– EPTfe - monofilament (Gore-tex)
– Polyester - braided (Ethibond)

Absorbable:

– Surgical - gut
– Plain gut - monofilament (30 days)
– Chromic gut - monofilament (45-60 days)

Synthetic:

– Polyglycolic - braided (16-20 days)
(Vicryl; Ethicon)
(Dexon; Davis and Geck)
– Polyglecaprone - monofilament (90-120 days)
(Monocryl; Ethicon)
– Polyglyconate - monifilament (Maxon)

Suture	Indications	Size	Needle	Absorption
Surgical silk	General closure of most oral soft tissues. Where non-resorbable suture, is not required and strength is required.	3/0 4/0	Cutting	Is completely degraded by two years Is a braided material and not as clean as new material.
Surgical gut	Extraction suture	3/0	Cutting	Completely absorbded within 30 days. Effective strength for 2-3 days in the oral cavity Excellent for oral mucosal when longer life is needed.
Chromic catgut Plain catgut + (Chromic salt)	General closure Chromic salt make it resistant to resorption and increase resoprtion time.	4/0	Taper	Completely absorbed in 45-60 days. Provides excellent strength for up to 5 days.
Monofilament nylon	Large flaps For extra strength like a palate closure Skin closure	3/0 4/0 6/0	Cutting	Non-resorbable with 15-20% degradation Excellent tissue compatibility Very clean
Polyglycolic acid	Alveolar mucosal Attached gingiva	4/0 3/0 4/0	Taper cutting	Completely absorbed in 16-20 days. Provides excellent strength to the oral mucosa for two weeks. Has a tendency to accumulate plaque be cause of its braided nature.

Q.199. Out of correct contoured buccal surface for food deflection.

1. 1
2. 2
3. 3
4. 4

Ans. In this question, the diagram should have been given, but they did not give diagram perhaps they might have forgotten. The area for food deflection occur on that surface area of tooth at and above the area of maximum bulge or contour.

Q.200. Cavity preparation on which location of tooth will give rise to black class I cavity (Spot the location of caries to make black class I cavity preparation).

1. 1
2. 2
3. 3
4. 4

Ans. In this question the diagram should be given but they did not give diagram perhaps they might have forgotten.

Class I cavity occur on lingual surface of lower anterior teeth and occlusal surface of premolars and molars and occlusal two thirds of buccal and lingual surface of molars.